DR GOWRI MOTHA

& KAREN SWAN MACLEOD

gentle first year

the essential guide to
mother and baby wellbeing
in the first twelve months

HARPER
thorsons

To my parents, who are the best; to my boys, who make me want to be the best.

HarperThorsons
A division of HarperCollins*Publishers*
77–85 Fulham Palace Road
Hammersmith
London W6 8JB

The website address is www.thorsonselement.com

and *HarperThorsons* are trademarks of
HarperCollins*Publishers* Ltd

Published by HarperThorsons 2006

10 9 8 7 6 5 4 3

© Dr Gowri Motha and Karen Swan MacLeod 2006

Dr Gowri Motha and Karen Swan MacLeod assert the moral right
to be identified as the authors of this work

Text illustrations by Mell Vandevelde

A catalogue record for this book is
available from the British Library

ISBN-13 978-0-00-721305-4
ISBN-10 0-00-721305-0

Printed and bound in Great Britain by
Martins the Printers, Berwick upon Tweed

contents

foreword

It has taken me far too long to try to think of what to say about Gowri. How do you describe a lady who you feel changed your experience of giving birth, a woman who thinks of her mothers and readers as if they were her children, someone who you believe contributed to you and your child?

I honestly believe that Gowri is a one-off and I feel so lucky to have been able to learn from her great knowledge and affection. It is brilliant that everyone can now share the Gowri experience through her books: becoming aware that we are animals experiencing mother nature's magic, learning how to open your body to its journey ahead and to connect with the most amazing thing inside you – your little baby. Both before and after birth, Gowri teaches you to visualize what is going to happen to you, and to understand how to make that as easy as possible through diet, exercise and just taking the time to breathe and pause! Gowri taught me what was happening physically to me and my baby and she also opened my mind to what was happening spiritually.

There is so much information available to us now about how to optimize our pregnancy that we can almost forget that there'll be a baby at the end of it! It's as if the journey becomes the destination. And that journey has continued after my baby's birth as well. There is so much to absorb and learn in the first few months of becoming a mother, and I have been so grateful for Gowri's support and expertise. She had lots of tips for soothing the baby to sleep and her medical training meant that I could really trust her advice when he was out of sorts! But as much as anything, my greatest comfort was knowing that my post-natal recovery ensured that I could dedicate all my energies to being the best mother I can be.

I am sure that by reading this book you too will experience the Gowri phenomenon and enjoy the most important journey life can ever give you – the gentle first year.

Stella McCartney

introduction

a shared journey for mother and baby

At every birth, two people are born - a baby and a mother.
Ancient Indian wisdom

It's a common complaint that after nine months of getting seats on the bus and foot rubs by night, the mother is all but forgotten when the baby is born. She might have a sore perineum and afterpains, but this just can't compete for attention with the baby's patch of fuzzy hair and ten perfect toes. This sudden neglect has always seemed strange to me because in India, where I grew up, the birth is regarded as a rebirth for the mother too.

Motherhood reveals a woman's best self, ready to nurture and compromise for love of her child.

All new parents aspire to being and doing their best for their babies, and it's important to recognize the journey the mother has to take, as well as her baby. This fundamental oversight is repeated at many different cultural levels, and it's not just partners and new grandparents who are at fault. Have you noticed how most baby books take sides? Some empathize with the baby – tiny, exhausted and completely dependent upon you; others go with the mother – huge, exhausted and completely dependent upon the midwife. The principal ambition of this book is to tell both sides of the story, because you and your baby both have a lot of growing and learning to do in this first year.

Those of you who followed the programme in my first book, *The Gentle Birth Method*, will know I regard pregnancy as a shared journey between mother and baby, and that I use a variety of different techniques – such as visualizations and self-care – to promote deep bonding in utero. *The Gentle First Year* builds on this foundation by nurturing your emotions every bit as much as your body, and showing you how to do the same for your baby.

the importance of bonding

If these twelve months are a mountain you must scale together, the success of the climb rests on the preparation made at base camp.

Bonding underpins both my prenatal and postnatal programmes. I believe that the more you can do to cultivate it (massage, songs, eye contact, play), the more mother and baby will thrive. If these twelve months are a mountain you must scale together, the success of the climb rests on the preparation made at base camp. I believe that the best start for every mother and baby is an intensive and exclusive confinement period in what I call the 'red tent', which eclipses everything other than getting to know each other. And I'm not alone in thinking this – I've got the weight of history on my side too.

the red tent

Much of my first-year programme is rooted in this ancient postnatal concept. The red tent has been passed down from the nomadic communities of the Jacobi era in the Middle East and still exists in modified form in my native India. The red tent refers literally to the tent to which the women retreated during their menstrual flow. Men were prohibited from entering, and all duties – cooking, cleaning and sexual relations – were suspended until they re-emerged three or four days later.

Why is this relevant? Well, apart from being used for this monthly hiatus, the red tent was also a post-partum retreat, where the new mother and baby rested, recovered and were restored from the birth for 40 days. During this time, the mother did not come out of the tent, but literally fed and slept with the baby, and was massaged and tended to by the other women.

It is still customary in India for the expectant woman to stay at her parents' home from the 28th week (seventh month) of pregnancy, and then for three months after the birth. The mother rests in a specially designated room where she is nourished, nurtured and allowed to heal in much the same way as advocated by the ancients. I grew up seeing at first hand the restorative effects of such intensive post-partum care. It is my wish to prescribe to my mothers a unique, powerful – and empowering – postnatal programme, which integrates these philosophies of the red tent with mainstream medical practices.

creating a cocoon

Of course, for the Western lifestyle, a literal interpretation of the red tent confinement is unrealistic. Many mothers try to discharge themselves from hospital the day after the birth, so convincing them to stay in a room for three months is hardly a viable option. But what is relevant is the idea of 'cocooning' yourself, drawing a metaphorical curtain around you which shields you from the demands and pressures of daily life. Life is not normal in those first three months – your sleep is broken, your body may well feel battered and bruised, and you face great challenges as you ease your baby into this noisy, bright world. But recovery and discovery lie before you, and the bond you cultivate with your baby has the transforming power to change both your lives.

The wisdom behind the confinement of the red tent is to promote rest, recovery and deep bonding. My strongest advice to new mothers is to stay at home as much as possible – certainly for the first three weeks, ideally up to six weeks and, in my dreams, up to three months. But there invariably comes a time when the outside world must become part of your lives again, and although you might have to go out with the pram to do the weekly shopping, it's also lovely to go for a gentle walk around the park. When you do start to go out together, dab a drop of Australian Bush Flower remedies – such as Angelsworth or Fringed Violet or the easily available Rescue Remedy – on the baby's fontanelle. This will soothe the baby from the cacophony of outside stimulus and can become a comforting ritual on your first excursions together.

how this book will support you

I feel this book will have succeeded in its purpose if it helps you to receive physical assistance in the early weeks after the birth, and emotional support for the developmental and nurturing issues which come thick and fast in the first year. You will find that the emphasis of this book naturally shifts as the baby grows.

In the first three months, the principal issues are physical. We can, together, help treat and heal any specific trauma you may have suffered from the birth; advocate treatments that fine-tune your body's transition out of the pregnant state; as well as addressing and resolving your emotional issues surrounding the birth. For your baby, we can explore how to make him or her feel emotionally held and secure; advise physical treatments that eliminate any residual pressures from the birth;

boost natural immunity; and offer practical tips to help soothe, calm and settle your baby into deep slumber.

After navigating this intense healing period of the first three months, the emphasis moves to a more emotional plane, showing you and your baby how to enjoy each other. I am opposed to the hot-housing trend, which places undue pressure on early achievement, and firmly believe that babies thrive when nurtured by delighted and committed parents.

It's not the 'big' things that matter – like speaking French or sleeping through the night – but the delicious little gestures that convey love, security and comfort.

To paraphrase John Lennon, 'Life is what happens to you whilst you're busy making other plans,' and there couldn't be a better sentiment for parenting. It's not the 'big' things that matter – like speaking French or sleeping through the night – but the delicious little gestures that convey love, security and comfort. A cashmere teddy bear may be intended as a big show of love, but a bedtime massage feels just as blissful to your baby; what's more, it is profoundly bonding and can become a much-loved part of your daily routine. So find the extraordinary in the ordinary, and look for joy – not perfection – in the details.

If having a baby takes away many things – freedom, independence, sleep, seats on the bus – it also gives back so much more: a sense of wonder, bold curiosity, seeing the world with fresh eyes again. A rebirth, perhaps!

PART ONE
recovery

the first week

embracing motherhood
bonding with the baby

She knew very well how babies smell; she knew precisely. 'Well,' the wet nurse began. '... They don't smell the same all over, although they smell good all over. Their feet, for instance, smell like a smooth warm stone, or like fresh butter ... And their bodies smell like a pancake that's been soaked in milk. And their heads, up on top, at the back of the head, where the hair makes a cowlick ... here is where they smell best of all. It smells like caramel. Once you've smelled them there, you love them whether they're your own or somebody else's.'
Perfume, Patrick Suskind

Having delivered thousands of babies over the years, one of my favourite moments is watching the new mother smelling her newborn baby's head for the first time. Most are hardly aware they're doing it, but in that split second when the mother inhales the exquisite scent of new life, she falls in love. After nine long months, she can at last see her baby, touch her baby and hear her baby, but it's when she smells her child's pristine dewiness that the cocktail of bonding hormones really starts to fizz. And it's not just a temporary kick. Years later, mothers can be found wistfully sniffing talcum powder bottles in supermarket aisles and wearing talc-based perfumes (astute perfume houses cottoned on to our nostalgia long ago).

Happily, it's a requited love. Whilst it takes weeks for the baby to decipher faces and sort out voices (everything sounds muffled in the womb), a newborn infant can detect the smell of her mother's milk almost immediately. It has been shown that a minutes-old baby, placed on the mother's tummy, will grapple, heave, shake her head from side to side, nuzzle into the mother's breast and find the nipple to suckle, led entirely by smell.

It's an amazing thing to see in action. At every birth I attend, I'm always looking for that transforming moment when the fundamental survival instinct and urge to protect becomes something deeper and more spiritual; an impulse that takes a parent beyond the instinct to merely raise a child to maturity, and actually nurture, cherish, indulge and adore the child to its best possible self.

We all know this as bonding, of course, the pop-psychology buzzword for the modern parent. But whilst bonding is indeed an inherent part of parenthood, we don't always acknowledge that it is not an automatic response. If you want a deep, nourishing relationship with your child which soothes your soul, then it will need tender cultivation, shared experience and, yes, a smattering of hormonal alchemy.

There's a line in Lucy Atkins' book, *Blooming Birth*, which really resonates with me: 'Birth is just the start – parenting's the biggie.' She's absolutely right, and the biggest help you can have when negotiating the myriad minefields of toddlerhood, pre-pubescence and adolescence is the solid bond you establish with your child during your pregnancy and at birth. Bringing with it an empathy, sensitivity and kindness that endure throughout the myriad experiences life throws at you, it starts right here, with your newborn and her soft, fuzzy head.

why bonding matters

The endorphins released mutually by mother and baby during the birth process are very important for the deep bonding and mutual attachment necessary for the survival of the infant. This is one of the reasons why I work so hard to deliver gentle births that will promote greater levels of endorphins being released at birth. In the interests of mother-child bonding, health professionals should be geared towards preventing fearful births where the fear hormone, adrenaline, inhibits endorphin production.

sleep bonding

My Mother came to me and lay down beside me, and the warmth of her body comforted me. Secure in the knowledge of her love, I began to cross over into sleep.
The Red Tent, Anita Diamant

The bonding power of sleep is profound. Sleep is the ultimate surrender, when we are most vulnerable, and it's impossible to attain if we do not feel relaxed, safe and warm. As adults we wouldn't dream of sleeping with – or even near – someone we didn't like or trust, and it's very much the case with babies too.

In every respect, you are your baby's protector. I am a firm believer in the emotional and physical benefits of mother and baby sharing a room – if not necessarily a bed – in the early weeks. Hailing from the red tent culture, I have seen at first hand the evident security this arrangement bestows upon the child. After all, having spent nine months drowsily curled up in the womb listening to the regular thud of your heartbeat, the immediate touch, sight and smell of you, the slumbering mother, is the next best thing to those warm, cosy waters. For mothers and fathers too, there is no greater sense of joy and peace than when their baby is blissfully asleep in their arms.

Shared sleep is indicative of shared love, and if you find that you can sleep through the grunts, snuffles, chatters and snores of a sleeping baby, then there is nothing more wonderful.

BEDSIDE CRIBS

A crib next to the parents' bed is the ideal scenario in my opinion; or even better, a bedside cot with one side that opens out completely to annexe to the mother's side of the bed. These save the mother from climbing out of her warm bed (especially in the cold, dark winter months), and she can easily slide the baby back into the safety of the cot's confines after the feed. All the big baby chain stores like Mothercare and John Lewis sell these bedside cots, but check the height before you buy. The height of the cot may not be compatible if you have, say, an iron or a sleigh bed.

BED SHARING

Sharing a bed is a trickier issue. In principle, it seems the most natural option, but that doesn't mean it's the safest – there have been various tragic incidents in which the mother or father has inadvertently smothered the baby in their sleep. Alcohol, drugs, medication and extreme exhaustion are all risk factors, but there have even been instances when the baby has been suffocated by the mother's milk-swollen breasts. UNICEF and the Royal College of Midwives recommend no co-sleeping under three weeks of age. The advice I give to my mothers is to share a room, not a bed, with the baby at night.

Case History: Karen and Ollie

I had read all the books saying not to rock/feed/carry your baby to sleep but Ollie was a restless baby, and in the early weeks that was the only way I could get him off to sleep. Still, by the time he was about eight weeks old, I knew I had to start to teach him to sleep without relying on stimulus from me. So, at his morning and afternoon nap, I began to lie on the bed with him. I turned him away from me so that he wouldn't think he was getting a feed, and would curl my arms and legs around him, with the top of his head nuzzled under my chin, and just the feel of my body, my warmth and my smell to reassure him.

For the first couple of attempts to put him to sleep, he cried for up to 40 minutes on and off, which was pretty hard to bear. But I stuck with it and very soon he understood that when we lay down together, he was just going to have a little sleep. I didn't sleep with him at night, so it was absolutely blissful to share that 30-minute nap with him in the day. We both slept so heavily - I'm sure our pheromones must have knocked each other out - and it kept me going at that point when the broken nights were really beginning to take their toll.

Strangely, I would always wake about 30 seconds before he did; he never once woke me up. I could actually hear his breathing change once I started to stir. When I moved him to sleep in his cot, a month later, he was absolutely fine about it and went straight to sleep without crying, but I still needed the naps too - my husband jokes that he sleep-trained me, rather than the other way round! But I'll always treasure our baby naps together. I'm convinced they contributed to the powerful bond between us.

BABY HAMMOCKS

In India it is traditional to tie a sari lengthways as a long, low-slung hammock from a ring on the ceiling, so that the baby is suspended about 30 inches above the floor. The sari tied in this way is called a *thottil* ('cradle') in southern India. The *thottil* creates a soft cotton sling for the baby, rather like the one depicted on birth announcement cards showing the baby being carried in a sling by a stork. Sometimes, a long piece of cotton can be used to tie the *thottil* instead of a sari. This is called a *dhoti*, which men wear like a sarong. The baby feels very comfortably held within this soft cotton sling. It allows good circulation of air, and deep sleep is promoted by the baby's spontaneous movements that rock the cradle.

Mothers who work in the fields in India resourcefully tie a sari onto the branch of a tree to create a cradle, and place their infant within. It is common for tourists travelling through India to be charmed by the sight of babies hanging in *thottils* from the trees!

The *thottils* are most commonly used in villages and in traditional families, but rocking cradles made of cane are also the prized possessions of many mothers. My mother had a rocking cradle for me and my siblings. I remember her rocking my youngest brother to sleep, and I often crept into the room to rock the cradle.

And it's not just an Indian tradition. The Mexican culture has historically endorsed hammock sleeping too, and now Australia is following suit. Neonatal units there have studied the positive effects of babies sleeping in baby hammocks and have reported many positive benefits, particularly better quality sleep. Mainly this is because of emotional security, as the baby feels snug and held, as if the sling is an extension of the womb or loving arms. But head support – and comfort – seems to play a role too. In particular, it was noted there was a dramatically reduced incidence of Flat Head Syndrome, a phenomenon increasingly seen in the West as a result of neonatal advice that babies must only be laid on their backs. I do not contradict this advice at all, but I do advise those mothers whose babies show signs of developing Flat Head Syndrome to place them in a hammock or *thottil* for a couple of hours each day. I recommend buying a baby hammock from www.babyhammocks.com as these have passed all safety checks.

SEPARATE ROOMS

London is a city of lanky Georgian and Victorian terraces, and I inwardly despair when I hear my London mothers relate their middle-of-the-night stories with the baby ensconced on an entirely different floor in the house. Not only is the baby isolated, but also the poor, exhausted mother is trudging up and down several flights of stairs each time the baby stirs. Some of my mothers consider this the easier option, however, and I do sympathize when they say they simply cannot sleep in the same room as their baby. Hormones are running at such a state of high alert anyway that every whisper and sigh their baby emits can drag them out of sleep and leave them permanently exhausted. This is no good to anyone and can compromise the quality of the mother's milk.

If you do choose to place your baby in a separate room, there is still plenty you can do to make sure the baby feels secure:

- Respond to the baby's waking cries quickly. She needs to see you and smell you as soon as she can, as this will reassure her that you are always at hand when she needs you.
- For the first few weeks, put the baby to sleep in a swinging crib or place the baby's Moses basket inside the big cot, beneath the mobile.
- When the baby has outgrown the Moses basket/crib (by around twelve weeks) put the baby to sleep in the big cot, under the mobile, which by now should be familiar.
- Place the baby to sleep on a baby sheepskin. These really do comfort babies, making them feel held, and they seem to sleep more soundly on them. The baby sheepskins are sheared to an extra-short length but, if you like, you can place the sheepskin under the baby's cot sheet.
- To make the big cot seem smaller, roll up two clean cellular pram blankets and lay them either side of the baby's waist, like mini bolsters. These help the baby feel more secure and confined, again echoing the womb. Equally, you can buy special baby mats, which have attached bolsters at the sides.
- Another tip is to roll a larger cellular cot blanket lengthways and loop it in a U shape. The U-bend should pat up against the baby's bottom, with the baby's legs hanging bent over the blanket and the blanket running up the baby's sides. This really helps the baby to feel held.
- If you have a cuddle cloth, tuck it next to your skin in your bra so that it absorbs your smell. Then you can tie this to the cot and help reduce any separation anxiety.

SWADDLING

One of the hardest things for the new parent – particularly the new dad – is getting used to the tiny proportions of the newborn body. An adult's big hands and strong arms can easily feel clumsy when that little body is flailing and wriggling about. But swaddling can really minimize that awkwardness. Swaddling is an age-old custom that crosses nearly every

gentle first year

culture in the world – from Eskimo babies in sealskins, African babies in *kakoi* slings to Japanese babies swaddled into the silken folds of *obi* wraps. Swaddling is fantastic for helping a baby feel secure. Keeping the arms and legs bound in a secure wrapping mimics the confines of the baby's beloved womb. When the baby is born, one of the most pronounced birth reflexes is the Moro, or startle reflex, when the baby suddenly throws out her arms and legs when startled. The Moro reflex is an involuntary response to threat and acts as the earliest form of 'fight or flight' response. This is generally more pronounced in boys than girls, and begins to fade away gradually from three weeks. It can be alarming for the baby who, at this point, has no idea that those flailing arms and legs are actually her own and often scratches herself, hence the need for scratch mittens.

I recommend swaddling the baby in a cellular cotton blanket for the first three weeks to give her the feeling of the continuity of being held in a womb. After this time, the baby usually starts to wriggle out of it. You can then move on to swaddling the baby under the arms so that the body and legs feel held but her arms can stretch out. After a couple of days of contented sprawled sleeping, the baby is ready to go into the now-popular baby sleeping bag.

---

note

Only ever use a cellular blanket for swaddling, as the intrinsic holes within the cellular blanket will provide a crucial air supply should the blanket go over the baby's face. The risk of this increases as the baby gets bigger and stronger, as the increased wriggling dislodges the blanket off the shoulders and moves it up around the face, risking suffocation.

---

the first week

how to swaddle

1 Take a cellular blanket and fold one corner up to the opposite corner, making a triangle.

2 Place the triangle so that the longest straight edge is arranged at the top.

3 Lay the baby down on the centre of the blanket, with her shoulders just an inch or so below this long edge.

4 Check that the lip of the blanket doesn't protrude so high above the shoulders as to cover the baby's mouth when she turns her head to the sides.

5 Take one corner from the right or left (whichever is shortest, depending upon how centrally you've placed the baby on the blanket) and snugly wrap it around the baby's body. Make sure the baby's arm is placed down at the sides, and pull the blanket down and around so that the corner can be tucked under the baby's bottom. Keep the tuck as flat as possible so it's not bulky and uncomfortable beneath the baby's body.

6 Pull over the remaining corner – again in a downward direction, with the baby's arm down at the corresponding side, and tuck under the baby's bottom. Again, keep the tuck as flat as possible.

a new way to handle babies

A new school of thought amongst maternity nurses in Los Angeles promotes extremely gentle and slow handling of babies. The traditional way to pick up babies is to lift them up to you and then bring them in close, but this new method involves bringing the baby in close to you *before* lifting them through the air.

water bonding

A lot of baby bonding is about summoning the sensations and security of the womb, and much of that can be re-created in water. I have long been a proponent of water births, believing them to be a more gentle transition for the newborn from the womb to the outside world. But even after the birth event itself, I often use water to soothe unsettled babies. One of the joys of my practice is giving cranio-sacral treatment to a baby while in a warm and safe baby pool.

THE DIVE REFLEX

Nine months in the amniotic fluids equips babies with a diving reflex, which is very strong at birth but fades over the following months as they rapidly adapt from a watery to an airy environment. Babies are fully capable and relaxed when momentarily submerged; their pronounced dive reflex kicks in and they hold their breath automatically. Try it yourself – if you blow onto your baby's face, you'll see she automatically holds her breath.

Test your baby's dive reflex by blowing onto her face. You'll see she automatically holds her breath.

BABY SWIM CLASSES

The dive reflex can be retained if the baby is exposed to water submersion on a regular basis. It would be wonderful if you could find a specialist baby swim class (I recommend them from four months onwards – see Resources). As well as keeping up the dive reflex, the best of these classes also place a strong emphasis on baby water safety – teaching them how to turn in the water, float on their backs (and therefore, breathe!) and how to hold on to the side should they fall into a pond or pool.

It's natural that you might feel apprehensive at the thought of your baby going under water, but you'll be surprised at how much she loves the feeling of weightlessness – it's the only time her little body is fluid and synchronized! She may well come up with her eyes wide and smiling, as babies don't shut their eyes underwater.

BATHTIME BONDING

On a smaller, more intimate scale, water bonding in the bath can play a part in your daily routine. My grandmother in India always said babies should be bathed before midday, not at night, as this closes off the chakras (the seven energy centres on the midline of the body) and inhibits vital growth and repair during sleep. If you can bathe your baby in the morning or at lunchtime, so much the better. However, I appreciate that this is not convenient for the Western lifestyle, where bathtime is often delayed until early evening when working mothers or fathers get home. The bonding opportunities bathtime presents are of course far more precious and must be respected. Equally, you may have another child who is already in an evening bathtime routine or is at school during the day and so can only bathe in the evening. If this is the case, a good compromise is to try and finish bathing before 6pm.

One to two drops of pure lavender essential oil mixed in with milk (so that it doesn't sit as a film on top of the water) and then added to the running water makes a lovely aromatic bath and will induce a gentle sleepiness just before bedtime.

A wonderful mother-baby bonding exercise is floating your baby on her back whilst maintaining eye contact. You can do this in the bath or in a pool (but if the pool has cool water, invest in a neoprene baby wetsuit - see Resources for details).

touch bonding

Of all the bonding methods, this has to be my favourite. Regular baby massage soothes the soul of every mother and child, and really forges a powerful empathy and trust between the two. I advocate daily baby massage and think the ideal time is immediately after the bath. No fancy oils are needed, just a good quality base oil such as extra virgin olive oil or sweet almond oil. Apart from the immunological and muscular benefits of the massage, these oils will really nourish and hydrate the baby's skin, which can look dry and flaky in the first few weeks after birth.

When using sweet almond oil, be sure to rule out any history of nut allergy. There has been a report that almond oil should be avoided if there is a history of epilepsy in the family.

If you would like to harness the benefits of aromatherapy for your baby, add just two drops of lavender essential oil to 50ml of your base massage oil. Lavender calms the central nervous system and is also a muscle relaxant.

I have devised these specific massage routines for you to use after bathtime. If you have followed my gentle birth method, some of the massage techniques will be familiar to you.

CREATIVE HEALING BABY MASSAGE

My method of baby massage is based on my knowledge of the creative healing lines of energy flow within the body. Creative healing was formulated and taught over half a century ago by Joseph B. Stephenson, a healer who devised a method of massage strokes that restored the energy flow within the body. Creative healing is now used widely in the United States and is beginning to filter over to Europe.

Some of the creative healing treatments are of special benefit for babies, such as the treatments for constipation and chest infections.

I appreciate that the creative healing method is more complicated than traditional baby massage, and I have produced a DVD (see Resources) which shows very clearly the baby massage routine. But in spite of my preference for this method, there really doesn't have to be a set formula when massaging your baby. The most important thing is loving, soothing, healing touch. Touch your baby with any of these intents and you will be amazed at the effect.

In the beginning, it may be hard to massage the limbs fully, as the baby will instinctively want to remain curled up into a little ball. But as you caress and stretch out those little arms and legs, you will be setting the baby on her first steps to standing tall and stretching high. And I defy anyone not to fall irrevocably in love with those peachy thighs, chubby arms and silky tender tummies! Your baby will delight in your spontaneous kisses whilst you massage her, and there will be a terrific endorphin rush for both of you.

basic instructions for creative healing massage

The limbs: Massaged in a downwards movement.

The abdomen: Massaged only in an upwards movement.

The back:

- The upper back is massaged upwards.
- The middle back is massaged sloping downwards.
- The lower back (sacrum) is massaged only in an upwards direction. The sacral nerves flow downwards like the roots of a tree, and it is physiologically sound to lift and reposition the nerve roots equally on both sides of the sacrum. This is done by massaging the sacrum lightly in an upwards direction only with the thumbs.
- While on the sacrum, performing very small arc-like movements with your thumbs over the little dimples for a few minutes a day can regulate your baby's bowels! If your baby is constipated, apply this very light massage for seven minutes. Make sure that your touch is very light so that you do not leave red patches on your baby's bottom!

The chest: The front of the baby's chest is massaged from the outer edges of the ribs converging inwards towards the breastbone (sternum). This movement also gets rid of congestion in the lungs, especially following a cough. Indeed, this movement prevents chest infections if the lungs are kept drained on a regular basis.

Routine: The first week just involves learning about your baby's body rather than initiating a formal routine. The guidelines above indicate the optimal directions for stroking different areas of the body – according to creative healing wisdom – but at this stage you just want the baby to respond positively to your touch and learn to find comfort in it. So touch your baby gently but confidently, and revel in the joy of touching your very own pristine, beloved baby.

You'll also find that getting to know your baby's body will empower you for when the baby becomes ill. It's easy to feel intimidated by the apparent fragility of those little bodies. With daily massage, however, you will know how yielding your baby's tummy is to regular touch and be able to identify when it is hard, distended or tender. Equally, you will instinctively learn the skin's natural colour and tone whilst you massage it, and therefore become more alert to rashes.

how massage increases baby's immunity

The constitutional benefits of touch are pre-programmed by Mother Nature. Every time you touch your baby, you create a virtuous circle whereby you pick up the bacteria living on your child's skin and pass it into your own system. Your adult system can easily develop antibodies against these bacteria that then pass into your breast milk, protecting your baby and boosting her own natural immune system.

Many of my mothers like to sing songs, rhymes and lullabies whilst they're massaging the babies, which is a lovely form of sound therapy. The classic songs 'You are my sunshine/My only sunshine' and *Summertime* are favourites, but I know some mums who swear by Don McLean's *Wonderful Baby*, not only because of the joyous baby-oriented lyrics, but also because of the many verses!

Best of all, maintain eye contact while you massage. Before you know it, your little butterball will be wriggling off to play some more and you'll consider yourself lucky to get her nappy on. So treasure these little rituals while you can and you'll have the memories to cherish forever.

I receive a lot of correspondence from mothers who follow the gentle birth method – either through my clinic or the book – and many of them stay in contact throughout the first year. Over the years, the tips I have received from these mothers have formed a massive store of information, some of which I will scatter throughout this book. Here is a collection of tips from Sonia Revelli, mother of four children.

Baby stretches to prevent colic. Sonia has found these to be invaluable and they can be done at every nappy change. However, avoid doing these immediately after a feed, as the baby may regurgitate.

Method
- Stretch the legs out first, then flex them at the knees and push the little thighs and legs back to the abdomen. Stretch and flex about four or five times.
- Then bring the little legs straight up and down by flexing both legs and extending onto the baby's tummy as much as possible. Repeat five to six times.
- Then cross the baby's ankles, left over right, and flex both thighs onto the tummy. Repeat by crossing the ankles, this time right over left.
- This becomes a lovely routine to do at all nappy changes.

Try not to breastfeed your baby lying down. Sonia feels that this predisposes the baby to getting glue ear, due to milk tracking up the Eustachian tube, which joins the ear to the throat.

If the baby has a cold, you might find the 'Mouche-Bébé' nose-blow device very useful. A French invention, it is a suction device with a reservoir which you can use to suction the nasal passages to aid breathing, and help the baby to sleep (see Resources for details).

If your baby has a chest infection, try using Moxa sticks. Cover the baby's legs with a cotton cloth so the skin isn't heated directly. Gently warm the outsides of the baby's legs with heated Moxa sticks, held at a safe distance from the baby's skin. Move the sticks up and down. This is amazing at clearing the nasal passages and lungs. [Moxa sticks are used in Chinese medicine and have excellent success rates. I use them a lot on pregnant mothers with breech babies. They have a 77 per cent success rate in turning the baby.]

TOUCH BONDING FOR PREMATURE BABIES

Touch bonding is never more important than with premature babies. How much you can lay on hands is, of course, determined by how early the baby came. But even if your child is in an incubator, there is still so much you can do to communicate and build a bond. For some parents, their child is so tiny the mother's little finger dwarfs the baby's hand, but no matter how small the baby, her instinct will still be to hold on to that finger as tightly as she can. In fact, it is months before babies develop the ability to actually let go, so you can maintain physical contact – albeit limited – for as long as you both want to.

Another comforting touch is placing the flat of your hand on the baby's tummy, avoiding the umbilical stump. Your warmth and the weight of your hand will be registered by the baby's body, and there's even evidence that suggests the baby will recognize the hand as yours – doctors have found that unborn babies kick more vigorously when their father's hand is placed on the mother's bump, as opposed to, say, the doctor's, so there'll be even more recognition with direct skin-to-skin contact.

Stroking the 'Third Eye'

Try very gently stroking the area between the eyebrows in a downwards direction – stroking downwards is very sedating. This space relates to the 'third eye', and stroking it can invoke deep mental relaxation. In Ayurveda, there is a renowned massage which involves pouring warm oil onto the third eye for up to an hour. It is noted for bringing about a profound sense of peace, and I have found this to be true for the modified stroking variation I use to settle fractious babies and to calm anxious pregnant mothers.

Stroking the Aura

You could also gently mould your hand in a cup shape around your baby's head and stroke her hair with your thumb. Then move your hand up to an inch away from the baby's head and make a series of long strokes, starting from the nose and sweeping to the back of the head or as far as you can go. This method, where you do not need to actually touch the baby's head, makes it ideal to calm premature babies. This is known as 'stroking the aura'.

You can also use this method to take the heat off the baby's head if you notice that her head is hot. Repeat as above, without touching the baby's head or neck, and stroke in one direction only as this flow is very relaxing for the baby.

Sceptical? If you relax and close your eyes and do it on yourself for a minute or two, you should be able to register an almost tingly sensation, like an electric current. Do this for about five to twenty minutes, or as long as you like. It's a loving, rhythmic sequence which can really get you involved with your baby's physicality, until such time as the baby is ready for full-on cuddles.

'Kangaroo Care'

When the baby can come out of the incubator for periods, take every opportunity to enjoy skin-on-skin touch. If you have been expressing your milk, you can now try direct breastfeeding. Equally, the father can try giving the baby a bottle of your milk. Both of you should try as much as possible to feed the baby without your shirts on as it's important that the baby can smell you and learn to associate your smell with loving touch. Remember, there are lots of bright lights around incubators – the baby may even have worn goggles – so she won't have terribly strong visual impressions of you. But she will have been able to smell you, so the closer she can actually get to you and your scent, the more relaxed she will be.

This intensive form of touch bonding is known as 'kangaroo care'. It has been proven to bring remarkable positive responses in premature babies. So take every opportunity to hold your baby against your chest. Let her smell your skin, nuzzle into your neck, sleep on your tummy, look up into your eyes. Don't put her down until the nurses are practically tugging her free. Every minute of skin-on-skin will make a difference.

Case History: Kangaroo Mother Care (KMC) for Premature Babies

This case history was contributed by paediatrician Dr G. Pramood Reddy MD DCH of the Fernandez Hospital for women and children in Hyderabad, India. The hospital was set up by my friend, Dr Evita Fernandez, whom I greatly admire for her dedicated work on the cutting edge of obstetric and neonatal care in India. It is Evita's – and my – wish that Kangaroo Mother Care is provided as an absolute necessity in developing countries where two-thirds of the world's low-birth-weight babies are born.

Rama Mani, a 35-year-old first-time mother, was treated for fertility issues for more than 14 years before she finally conceived. Unfortunately, during her pregnancy she suffered from many medical problems, including gestational diabetes, pre-eclampsia, fibroids and the problems that accompany an Rh-negative blood group! Despite the obstetric precaution of placing a cervical stitch to prevent premature labour, she went into labour at 30 weeks and delivered a baby girl weighing only 1.28kg. The baby was initially looked after in an incubator but as early as possible – by day 12 – she was moved to the Kangaroo Mother Care Ward.

Rama said that finally holding her baby next to her skin was one of the most joyous moments of her life. She was able to breastfeed her baby on demand and the baby gained weight notably faster than she would have if she were still in an incubator.

More importantly, Rama finally felt that she was able to nurture and mother her baby, and she confidently took her daughter home less than three weeks after the birth. Rama was so fascinated with the concept of Kangaroo Mother Care that she made her husband carry the baby around as well! Subsequently her daughter thrived and, despite her uncertain start to life, progressed rapidly to catch up with her full-term peers.

play bonding

Babies learn through play, but they also love through play, and so do we. Playing is an intrinsic part of bonding because to play with your baby is to delight in what she can do. There is no sophistication in baby play – no cultivated wit or superior irony – only the unbridled joy that comes with achievement and the thrill of the new. It is obvious, naïve, heartfelt and worn on the sleeves of both her babygro and your jumper.

Toys are great educational tools for the early months, but contact play – such as tickling or raspberry blowing – boasts benefits beyond the immediate joy of close touch. The skin is an organ which is stimulated by touch. The skin's nerve centre, the brain, releases a rush of feel-good hormones called endorphins every time you squeeze, stroke or tickle your baby. In fact, there is mounting evidence that deprivation of touch in childhood can actually reprogramme the brain and contribute to antisocial behaviour in later life. So getting physical when you play with your baby has far-reaching benefits, as well as boosting self-esteem and making you both feel good.

The skin's nerve centre, the brain, releases a rush of feel-good hormones called endorphins every time you squeeze, stroke or tickle your baby.

You can't help but clap with delight as your baby builds her first tower; both giggle helplessly when you tickle her on the changing mat, and revel in the excitement when your baby does a 'boo' to your 'peek'. Playing is like smiling when you're sad – it instantly makes you feel better. Each time you play with your baby, the world is new to you again, fresh and waiting to be explored. So turn every waking moment into an opportunity to share a giggle or show something new. Each time you do, your soul is renewed, your heart grows larger and your love becomes deeper.

breastfeeding

By rights, the issue of breastfeeding should be included in the 'bonding' section, as it is one of the most profoundly intimate and loving exchanges between mother and baby. The physical skin-on-skin contact helps the baby still feel closely connected to the mother's body, which has protected and nurtured the baby during the pregnancy. This feeling of security cannot be underestimated as the baby has, of yet, no sense of being physically separate from its mother. To the baby's limited sense of self, they are one person, and breastfeeding helps enormously in preserving that security. For the mother too, breastfeeding acts as a halfway house, as she adjusts to the physical separation from her child, which is, of course, the necessary result of birth.

From a practical point of view breast is best and easiest, and it's always just the right temperature. It is easily digestible, organic and, best of all, free! Plus, it helps the mother regain her figure more quickly. Breastfeeding burns approximately 500 calories a day. The baby's sucks stimulate the release of oxytocin from the mother's brain – the hormone responsible for contractions in labour – helping the womb shrink back into the pelvis far more quickly, and the mother to lose tummy fat and get back into her jeans!

Of course, the nutritional benefits of breastfeeding are what we really want to shout about. As well as passing on vital antibodies, which boost the baby's immune system, a mother's breast milk is perfectly tailored to her baby's individual needs. There are so many health benefits to breastfeeding that they alone are most women's incentives to carry on:

benefits of breastfeeding

- Reduced incidence/severity of eczema and asthma, childhood diabetes, gastric, urinary and respiratory tract infections and ear infections
- Higher IQ
- Less likelihood of cardiovascular disease or obesity in later life
- Long-term breastfeeding (at least a year) can reduce the risk of several cancers, such as ovarian and pre-menopausal breast cancer
- La Leche League has reported that breastfeeding can protect from osteoporosis in later life.

the father's role in breastfeeding

Yes, fathers actually play a very important role in breastfeeding. Studies have shown that the father's attitude to breastfeeding can determine whether or not the mother begins and continues to breastfeed. If he is against it, it is usually a direct response in which he sees his partner's breasts as sexual organs and is reclaiming them for himself, especially if his partner didn't want her breasts to be touched during pregnancy. The father might also feel that the side-effects of breastfeeding – such as tiredness or low libido – puts too much pressure on the parents' relationship and ask for breastfeeding to be abandoned. If this is the case, try to negotiate a time frame you are both happy with, up to which you will feed. Stress to your partner that this is only a temporary stage and your hormones will return to normal after you have stopped feeding.

Even if your partner is fully supportive of you breastfeeding, it is still worth encouraging him to feed the baby as much as possible. You can easily express your breast milk so that the father can feed the baby and feel more involved in this aspect of nourishing and nurturing his baby.

the different stages

THE FIRST FEW DAYS

Breastfeeding changes with different stages. The first stage occurs in the first few minutes after birth until three to five days later, and is the real 'feed on demand' stage – the more sucking the baby can do in these early days, the more bountiful the milk supply. Some babies (particularly those born by Caesarean section), however, may be exhausted and sleepy after the birth, and the appetite centre in their brain may not switch on for as long as 48 hours after the birth. In this acute period, the baby feeds on colostrum – a thick, creamy-yellow first milk that is absolutely jam-packed with goodness. It is the most optimal food of a baby's entire life, quenching their thirst, filling their tummies for the first time (and so helping pass the meconium from their bowels) and equipping them with a hit of vitamins, minerals and antibodies which will last for up to six months. In the UK, 69 per cent of mothers begin to breastfeed after birth.

---

correct latch technique and tips

- Tummy to mummy: lay the baby across your lap, with the baby's tummy lying next to your tummy. The baby should be supported high enough so that her face is at breast height. A C-shaped breastfeeding pillow is ideal as it is long enough to curl around you, support the full weight of your baby and bring her up to the right height for you. This will help you to sit comfortably without having to bend over, preventing neck and upper back strain.
- Nose to nipple: Move the baby towards the breast and stimulate your baby's rooting reflex by brushing your nipple on your baby's upper lip. This will encourage the baby to open her mouth. (Never move your breast to the baby – it must always be the other way round.)

- When the baby's mouth is open very wide, place the baby on the breast so that her bottom lip is curled back and her chin is pressed into the lower breast area (her chin should touch the breast first). In ratio terms, her mouth should cover the areola above the nipple one part to three parts below the nipple.
- The nipple should be directed at the back of the mouth, as far away as possible from the baby's tongue, as the baby doesn't actually suck the nipple itself, but stimulates the wider areola for milk release (the NCT says pertinently: it's breastfeeding, not nipple-feeding).
- Sit centrally. This is vital for back care.
- If your baby is particularly windy, modify this technique by sitting the baby into a more upright position. Each time the baby naturally breaks off, wind gently.
- To break the latch, never just pull the baby off, as they get a powerful suction going! Put your little finger into the corner of her mouth first to break the suction.

Breast and Nipple Protection

In the early weeks, your breasts and nipples are naturally going to feel sensitive, even sore, until they adjust to breastfeeding. The most important preventative measure is to make sure the baby is latching on properly (see above). Some mothers like to use a barrier cream such as Lansinoh (which is pure lanolin) or Kamillosan after every feed for the first few weeks until you adjust. It is not strictly necessary to wash it off before the next feed, but I do advise it, as the commercial varieties do contain some preservatives.

An alternative way to treat sore nipples is to express and rub a little of your milk onto them and allow them to air dry. Equally, if the nipples are very bad, or bleeding, some midwives recommend applying Vaseline before putting on the lanolin barrier creams. I have had mothers swear by it. If your nipples are too sore to feed, latex or plastic nipple guards are available at most pharmacies and can tide you over for a few days whilst the nipple heals. But if it is getting to this stage, please see a breastfeeding counsellor or lactation consultant for advice. They may also recommend that you express your milk for a couple of days and feed from a bottle (remember to express 30–45 minutes before the feed is due, so that the baby is fed on time).

If your breasts feel hot and tender when engorged in the early days, savoy cabbage leaves from the fridge naturally cup the breast and provide an instant cooling balm, or just drape over a cold wet flannel. Equally, you can buy gel-pads that you leave in the freezer. They are breast-shaped and can be placed reasonably discreetly inside the bra.

Although it is normal to feel a slight sharpness in the early days, breastfeeding should be comfortable. If you experience any sharp 'cut glass' shooting pains (indicative of thrush, see page 303) or redness of the breast tissue, lumps or feverishness (indicative of mastitis, see page 292) see your breastfeeding specialist or health visitor immediately. Mastitis can be treated with Bowen treatments and massage (see page 30) or in some cases antibiotics. Thrush can be treated with antifungal creams/tablets.

massage technique for blocked milk ducts

The following light massage technique clears the breast lymphatics and reduces the incidence of blocked milk ducts and mastitis. Using the middle three fingers, gently massage in ever-increasing clockwise circles from the edge of the areola to the upper breast and armpit area. Perform eight to ten times, twice a day.

bowen technique for all grades of mastitis

Bowen moves can be performed around the breast in an elliptical pattern, and I can vouch for the fact that mothers experience almost immediate relief. You can treat yourself whenever you feel your breasts are becoming sore or engorged.

THE SECOND STAGE

After three to five days (usually five days for Caesarean mothers), when most of the placental hormones (oestrogen and progesterone) have left the mother's body, prolactin is produced and the main milk 'comes in'.

Most textbooks on breastfeeding explain that the breast milk flows in two stages: the fore milk and hind milk. Whilst I respect this viewpoint, I reject the concept that there are two types of milk. I am also sceptical of rigid feeding times in the first two weeks. Some babies are better than others at breastfeeding, and their skill can make a big difference to how long a feed takes. Another important factor is how quickly the mother 'lets down' her milk. Again, some are faster than others, which determines how long the baby is on the breast. I therefore advise my mothers to relax if their baby stays on an individual breast for just 20 minutes.

Breastfeeding Problems in the Second Stage

This second stage of breastfeeding is characterized by engorgement and leaky nipples, and mastitis is most common at this point. This is because it takes a few weeks for the milk supply to even out. Mastitis occurs when residual milk becomes compacted and the surrounding tissues inflamed. If you suffer from mastitis but are leaving the baby on for 40 minutes or more, check the baby's latch (see box, page 27). Poor latch technique is incredibly common and can lead to prolonged and inefficient feeding. Sometimes the difference between a good and poor latch can be a matter of millimetres, so I strongly recommend seeing a specialist/counsellor at a breastfeeding clinic who can analyse and correct your latch. (Your midwife/health visitor will be able to give you details of your local clinic.)

Mothers sometimes get into a habit of feeding their baby in one position, or they favour one side over another. Vary your routine, but always start each feed on the same side you finished the previous feed. Some mothers keep a notebook next to their feeding chair to remind themselves of whether it's left or right this time, but you can also try reminding yourself by pinning a ribbon around the front clasps on your breastfeeding bra or wearing a hair band on the corresponding wrist. I laugh that you can always tell the more practised breastfeeding mothers – they're the ones who absent-mindedly cup their breasts (one side will be heavier than the other) or gently press the upper breast area in the café or in the park. They become so fine-tuned to the subtle difference between breast swell and heaviness, they check their breasts unconsciously!

Introducing a Feeding Routine

This is also the time to introduce more of a feeding routine, rather than baby-led demand feeding. I recommend a schedule of feeding every three to four hours in a 12-hour day. I have noticed that when babies are introduced to breastfeeding within an hour of birth, they naturally seem to want to feed at more regular intervals and sleep for longer intervals between feeds.

THE THIRD STAGE

By four months, into the third stage, the leaky nipples and feeling of engorgement/heaviness have gone. It is common for many mothers to think their milk supply is drying up and so stop breastfeeding. This is usually an incorrect assumption. Often the lack of engorgement is just a case of the milk supply being highly regulated – both in quantity and timing – as the breasts adapt very quickly to their natural role. They're still full, just not swollen. It's worth remembering during this 'doubting' period that breast milk provides all the nutrition that most infants need up to six months of age, and that it is still the best option for your baby. Unfortunately, this advice tends to fall on deaf ears, as in the UK only 28 per cent of mothers are still breastfeeding by four months, and 21 per cent by six months.

Breast milk provides all the nutrition that most infants need up to six months of age.

Bear in mind, too, that milk supply is a question of mental attitude. Milk is produced by the hormone prolactin and is let down by the hormone oxytocin, both of which are regulated by the pituitary gland in the brain. So although milk comes from the breast, it is controlled by your brain. If you believe in your ability to produce milk and wholeheartedly want to carry on breastfeeding, you will produce sufficient milk.

If you are worried about your milk supply, consider using an electric pump (so much better than the manual ones) very gently for 15 to 30 minutes at the end of the day. You may well have scarcely any milk (1–2oz) at this time for the first few days but that will very quickly build up as your body responds to the new demand. Also, keep an eye on your diet, particularly once you start weaning (from four to six months) and begin to drop feeds. That is the most dangerous time for breastfeeding as the reduced number of feeds is registered as less demand by the brain, so less milk will be produced. Avoid skipping meals (in fact you must try to eat up to 500 calories more, each day). Drink at least two litres of water per day and avoid alcohol. Exercise only gently and rest/sleep properly. You'd be amazed at what effect tiredness has on milk production!

how to make great milk

WHAT TO EAT

The hormones in your body naturally make milk after birth (even whilst you sleep), but quality control is your responsibility. Those of you who followed the gentle birth method will be used to a fairly controlled diet. If you are new to the gentle way, this may come as something of a shock: I advocate a sugar-free, wheat-free diet during pregnancy to moderate the weight gain of both mother and baby, and minimize fluid retention.

For at least the first month after birth (and longer if they can bear it), I encourage my mothers to stick to their antenatal diet but for quite different reasons. In the womb, your baby will have ingested what you ate, and so have become accustomed to your dietary tastes. After birth, your milk will be uniquely and subtly flavoured according to your preferences, and it is my personal belief that many instances of colic/wind in babies can be attributed to the mother's sudden change in dietary habits.

You can go for a low-wheat, rather than no-wheat diet, and keep sugar to a minimum – but rather than thinking about restrictions, you should try to think about what your diet can do for your milk.

Try to think about what your diet can do for your milk.

The way to view it is that until the baby is fully weaned, breastfeeding is, to all intents and purposes, another segment of pregnancy – your baby is still as dependent on you for nourishment as she was *in utero*. Of course, watching your diet is another sacrifice for you, and after nine long months of pregnancy and a tiring birth, you may well have had enough, but you're on the home straight, and this is a relatively short period of time in the grand scheme of things.

Foods to choose:
- Small fish (high in omega fats) such as sardines, kippers and herrings
- Lean proteins
- Vegetables
- Oats
- Salads
- Fruits
- Lots of water (room temperature)

This will create a nourishing, rich milk upon which your baby will both thrive and settle. I think that poor-quality milk is a prime suspect in fractious, irritable babies.

FISH SOUP AND GREAT MILK

In the tropics where I grew up, the fisherwomen's baskets were full of small coin-like fish, or little elongated fish or sardines. They were all grouped together under the common name *podimeen*, which literally means 'small fish'. I distinctly remember my grandmother advising my mother to make a light soup of these fish and consume it daily to improve the quality and quantity of breast milk to feed my younger siblings. Perhaps you could modify a suitable recipe from your cookbooks at home to take whilst breastfeeding?

Something I recommend highly, but which is quite a cultural departure for most of my mothers, is the postnatal pudding, *raagi kallie* (a common name for a nutritious pudding or paste). In southern India, this pudding is made from a grain called *raagi* ('finger corn' in English), but you can make *kallie* using ground millet grains.

Recipe for Raagi Kallie

Take a cup of powdered grain and add to a pint of boiling water in a saucepan on the hob. Stir the mixture all the time. As it begins to thicken, add two tablespoons of ghee (clarified butter) and a tablespoon of powdered jaggery (palm sugar) till the whole mixture takes on the consistency of firm dough.

The end product is warm, moist and very tasty – little wonder that it's an intrinsic part of the immediate post-partum programme in India. Formulated especially for the needs of the new, breastfeeding mother, it contains high levels of calcium, protein, fat and carbohydrate, which all provide amazing nutrition for good breast milk production. Of course, you'll have precious little time to make this yourself, so following the red tent concept (see page x), ask someone close to make it for you. You may feel like this is another favour to ask other people to do for you, but people always want to help when there's a new baby and I'm sure your partner, mother, best friend or doula would be delighted to make it for you during the first two weeks after the birth. The ingredients themselves are cheap and can be easily found at larger supermarkets or at Asian grocers (I found jaggery at Tesco).

So your diet should be optimal, and so should your fluids. Keep off alcohol, especially spirits, but if manners or sanity dictate accepting a small tipple, limit it to one small glass of wine on very special occasions. If you can't completely give up tea or coffee, please at least give up coffee and drink just cups of weak tea – but if your baby is unsettled or windy, you'll have to come off it altogether. Herbal and green teas are ideal. Many midwives swear by fennel/nettle tea for reducing wind/colic/fretfulness in babies. Please remember to drink at least two litres of water per day, as hydrating yourself will boost your milk volume and quench your baby's thirst. Keep a bottle of water next to your feeding chair and another next to your bed so that it's always to hand – many mothers report a mad thirst as soon as they begin a feed.

PROBIOTIC SUPPLEMENTS

As with the gentle birth method, I advise you to top up your diet with probiotics to help encourage the growth of friendly bacteria in your gut and prevent thrush (which is very common in the first week after birth). And a supplement of digestive enzymes will ward off indigestion and prevent bloating, both of which are problems due to the massive hormonal shifts after birth. By extracting every morsel of goodness from your diet, these supplements will help boost the quality of your milk; and by eliminating wind from your digestive system, the milk you pass on to your baby should be correspondingly flat.

EXERCISE

Strenuous exercise should be avoided for the first few weeks, certainly the first three, and ideally introduced after six weeks. This is because your body is still tired from the birth and trying to recover. You will probably find that you are losing a lot of weight in these first few weeks anyway and added exercise could have a big effect on your milk production, especially in the early days. Your body needs an extra 500 calories per day just to breastfeed (that's more than double the excess you needed during pregnancy) so do conserve your calories, or the quality of your milk will suffer.

COMPLEMENTARY THERAPIES

If you think your milk supply is low by the end of the first week, homeopathy can really help your milk come in. I recommend the following, three times a day for three days:

- Sepia 30c – If you are exhausted
- Cocculus 30c – If you are exhausted with broken sleep
- China 30c – If you are exhausted from breastfeeding

I also prescribe to the mothers at my clinic a homeopathic remedy that supports breastfeeding. I source this remedy from a revered 95-year-old homeopath in India. The formula decidedly improves the quality of breast milk and is great for the early days during transition from colostrum to more copious quantities of breast milk. He has named it Lactors and the remedy includes Calc flour 6c, Lecithin 6c and Asafoetida 6c (see Resources for details).

Reflexology has long been known to improve lactation, and I always perform some reflexology on the new mothers at my clinic. It has now been formally trialled at one of the main teaching hospitals in London to see if it can improve breast milk production for mothers of premature babies, and the results were favourable. I hope this will mean a more widespread take-up of reflexology among postnatal health professionals such as midwives and health visitors, and at breastfeeding clinics.

Case History: Reflexology and Breastfeeding

One of my colleagues referred a mother of Asian origin to me, just one week after her baby was born. She was unable to produce any breast milk at all.

I prescribed deep reflexology three times a week, concentrating on the pituitary and hypothalamic reflex areas in the brain, as well as on the breast reflex and digestive areas. I also prescribed my favourite homeopathic remedy, Lactors, which improves breast milk production. Along with this I advised her to make a soup of small-boned fish like sardines or whitebait (see page 34). She was advised to pressure-cook the fish – to really pulp it so that the bio-available calcium could be extracted from the fish to help her lactation. I also recommended a daily drink made from an infusion of fennel seeds (see below).

Within a day she went from producing 10 drops of milk to 50. A day later she was up to 10ml and then again up to 20ml. Within two weeks she was breastfeeding satisfactorily, even though she did supplement at night.

Recipe for Fennel Tonic

The Ayurvedic herbal tonic called Jeerarishtam is a boon to new mothers in India and improves lactation tremendously. The main ingredient of this preparation is fennel seeds, and for mothers who can't get hold of Jeerarishtam, then a simple recipe is to take a teaspoon of fennel seeds, boil it in half a pint of water, reduce it down to a cupful and drink this daily for three months after the birth.

The following postnatal milk-boosting recipes are Syrian in origin, and contributed by one of my favourite mothers, Rima Stait.

Recipe for Chicken Broth Porridge

1 whole chicken
5 cups of boiling water
Salt and pepper to taste
1 cup of Quaker Porridge Oats
Honey and a sprinkle of cinnamon

1 Cut the chicken into relatively small pieces. Place in a saucepan and cover with the boiling water.
2 Cover and boil for an hour. Season with salt and pepper to taste.
3 Allow to cool and remove all bones from the chicken, shredding the meat into bite-size pieces.
4 Boil the porridge oats with the remaining chicken broth (which should be about 4 cups) in the saucepan (without the chicken). Stir for 15 minutes over a low heat.
5 Add the chicken and stir occasionally for another 15 minutes.
6 Just before the end of cooking time, add honey and a sprinkle of cinnamon to taste.

NB You can substitute lamb off the bone for the chicken.

Recipe for Caraway Dessert

Traditionally this recipe is made by the grandmother, and it's a labour of love.

6 cups of boiling water
2 cups of sugar
1 cup of powdered rice
¼ cup of caraway powder (see Resources)
2 tablespoons of cinnamon
Mixed nuts (pistachios, almonds, walnuts, pine nuts ...)

1 Mix all the ingredients together in a saucepan, except for the nuts.
2 Leave to boil gently over a low heat for an hour, stirring continuously, until the mixture turns thick. (Thickness can be controlled by adding more boiling water if needed.)
3 Pour into small dessert glasses and refrigerate.
4 Soak the nuts in warm water for an hour and peel off any excess skin.
5 Remove the dessert from the refrigerator an hour or so before serving, as it is best eaten at room temperature. Sprinkle the nuts over each dessert glass.

emotional minefields

baby blues

One of the most oft-heard statements in the delivery room is: 'This is the happiest day of my life.' But I've long felt that statement has a lot to answer for because it implies that happiness is absolute, untainted by any other more complex emotions such as anxiety, anger or resentment. Three days later at home or on the postnatal ward when the baby blues kick in, it's usually a different story anyway! Whilst for many mothers the love for their baby is instant, deep and undeniable, for equally as many others, the maternal response is cautious, fearful and even apathetic.

As I wrote earlier in this chapter, bonding is neither automatic nor immediate. Even those mothers who reported a love-at-first-sight reaction will tell you that however powerful that thunderbolt, their love has grown infinitely deeper with the years. Initial ambivalence doesn't signify lack of maternal feeling – or, as some fear, psychosis – but rather a hormonal flux.

During your pregnancy, practically everything that can be measured and evaluated is recorded – blood pressure, sugar levels, volume of amniotic waters, size of the baby's tummy, the size of the fundus (your tummy!). And yet the catalyst for all this activity is the dramatic hormone change. During pregnancy, levels of the hormone oestrogen from the baby's placenta are 300 times higher than normal, while progesterone and relaxin levels are 30 times higher. During birth your body is flooded with oxytocin from your own hypothalamus and pituitary gland. After giving birth, the oestrogen and progesterone ebb away to allow for the greater flow of prolactin from your pituitary gland. The rigours of pregnancy and birth are small beer compared to these rocking hormone changes, so it's little wonder if you feel emotionally fragile.

Put frankly, it takes time to feel normal, and the immediate postnatal phase should come with a mental health warning! Fortunately, the mental and emotional aspect of birthing is becoming more understood. At antenatal classes, parents are told to expect the baby blues coming along with the milk, and any residual stigma or taboo surrounding postnatal depression has disappeared as we've learnt more about it. Postnatal depression does not mean a maternal vacuum – it's just chemistry.

Well, the first step is recognizing the symptoms and asking for help. In the first week after birth, extreme tiredness, apathy about the baby, loss of appetite, anxiety, insomnia, weepiness or desperation are all indicators of the baby blues and incredibly common. Fifty to eighty per cent of mothers experience one, or a range, of these emotions, so it's more likely that you will too. The cause is straightforward: the milk let-down hormone, prolactin, is present in ever increasing levels during pregnancy but surges in greater quantities once the main placental hormones – oestrogen and progesterone – have mostly been excreted after the birth of the baby and the expulsion of the placenta. This means a massive drop of oestrogen and circulating progesterone as well. This is like a hormonal cold turkey for the body and it takes a couple of days to readjust. Medically, it has become common practice to treat postnatal depression with a natural form of progesterone in large doses. I have found that rose otto oil massage really helps too, mostly because it is highly oestrogenic and is a safe source of plant oestrogens.

tips for beating the baby blues

I ask mothers to look in the mirror every morning and say out loud to themselves: 'I love my life' several times, maybe even 30 times! This feels strange initially but after a few days the programming kicks in and you really will feel better about your life. For milder cases of depression, I also encourage my mothers to sing - yes, really. To begin with, they often have to force themselves, as singing - like smiling - is naturally joyous. But it's a case of 'fake it till you make it'. The joy that comes from this small gesture is deeply underestimated and irrepressible - and your baby will love it too.

postnatal depression

Postnatal depression isn't quite so textbook as the baby blues. It can come on at any time up to a year after the baby is born. Many mothers feel more depressed at four to five months than in the first week, as the immediate post-birth euphoria is attributed to the endorphins that are released in great quantities during the birth process. Once the endorphin levels drop, the broken nights take their toll. Breastfeeding depletes the mother's fragile energy reserves, and the days can easily settle into a tedious, unending schedule of nappy changes, naps and feeds. This routine can be particularly tough on career-minded mothers.

Postnatal depression (PND) affects 15 per cent of mothers, which is still statistically significant. Symptoms include those of the baby blues (see previous page), compounded with:

- feelings of inadequacy
- despondency
- panic
- guilt
- mania
- no desire to breastfeed
- not caring about your appearance
- exhaustion
- headaches
- chest pains

Serious cases of PND are called postpartum psychosis and are fortunately rare (only one to two per cent of mothers are affected). Symptoms include severe mood swings and in some cases suicidal thoughts or thoughts of harming the baby. The mother may also experience hallucinations or confusion.

PND is an imbalance of the brain chemistry, but I always reassure my mothers that their hearts are still beating for their baby. An instant tonic, which can really elevate your mood, is an aromatherapy massage with rose otto essential oil. This contains many oestrogenic substances and is as therapeutic as it is luxurious. Rose otto works like a cerebral 'upper' to bridge the gap when hormone levels fluctuate, and it can have astounding results (see case history, page 45). Remember, communication can happen in many ways, and if conversation about your feelings is just too confrontational, allowing yourself to be massaged and touched will keep you connected to others and stop you withdrawing into yourself.

After the birth, fathers who have learnt creative healing techniques in pregnancy can use their skills and treat the mother to postnatal treatments. This will give the father a wonderful opportunity to maintain close physical contact with the mother when she needs physical and emotional comfort.

---

note

In all cases of post-birth blues, a good homeopath will help you find the appropriate remedies to help you work through your hormones and find your true emotions.

Case History: Rose Otto Oil Massage and Postnatal Depression

I remember very clearly a mother who was referred to me with clinical postnatal depression. She had stopped breastfeeding, had a very offhand attitude towards the baby, who was 10 days old, and her mother and husband had sought professional help when she had aggressively flung the baby onto the bed. The consulting psychiatrist wanted to hospitalize her when she was brought to me. I prescribed an aromatherapy massage with a massive dose of rose otto oil, much more than I would normally recommend. (Rose otto holds a higher concentration of the medicinal fractions of the rose oil.) She received a total body massage for a full hour, followed by some reflexology. I worked really intensively on relaxing her and making her feel cared for. The result was almost instant – even by the end of that first session, her demeanour changed and she seemed more interested in the baby, although she still wasn't allowed to handle him.

I asked her to come back every other day, and by the third session she had improved so much that she resumed breastfeeding under supervision. Her husband had taken a month off work to deal with the domestic crisis but was able to return after just over a week. Her mother stayed with her during the day so that the new mother felt supported, which gave her an ability to cope. I advised her to carry on daily with the rose otto massage (although at lower dosages) – either as self-massage or administered by her husband – to keep her mood lifted. And it worked – she never needed to come back to me again.

rose otto oil self-massage

1 Blend ten drops of rose otto oil into 20ml of base oil such as extra virgin olive oil or sweet almond oil.
2 Firmly apply to the arms and legs in long downwards strokes.
3 Apply to the upper half of the torso in an upwards direction in small clockwise circles, draining the tissue fluids over the neck and upper chest into the triangular area above the collarbone. (For those of you who have followed the gentle birth method, this massage follows the creative healing lines of drainage described there.)
4 The abdominal area is massaged in an upwards direction and the waist swept from the periphery to the central areas.
5 Repeat daily. Do not wash off the oil for at least four hours.

rose otto oil bonding tip

If you are performing the massage in the morning, and so wearing the scent during the day, the baby is going to associate rose scent with you. You might like to strengthen this connection and comfort the baby by burning rose oil or a rose-scented candle in the nursery. Or dab a drop of rose otto oil onto a piece of muslin and tie it to the side of the cot.

Recipe for a Good Postnatal Anti-depression Herbal Tea

½ teaspoon of raspberry leaves, dried
½ teaspoon of rosemary leaves, chopped
½ teaspoon of skullcap
½ teaspoon of liquorice, shredded

Add all the herbs to half a pint of boiling water. Allow to steep for twenty minutes, then strain and drink. Take this daily for about two months after the birth.

OTHER CAUSES OF PND
Poor Acceptance of Birth Experience

Postnatal depression primarily occurs from hormonal imbalance, but there are extenuating factors that can compound it, such as facing up to the birth experience (see 'Birth Acceptance', page 50). A whole host of feelings can complicate the mother's emotional landscape. These include disappointment with how they felt their bodies performed, anger, feelings of violation, frustration and even guilt.

You can start to accept the birth either by writing everything down, or talking it over with someone – be it your husband, mother, best friend, midwife or health visitor. You could even apologize to your baby if you feel that you might have resented being pregnant. Your baby will hear you and you will both feel released from tension. It sounds kooky, but you'd be amazed at the relief that can come from articulating pent-up guilt.

Case History: Julia and Felix — Accepting the Birth and Apologizing to Your Baby

I had to have a Caesarean with my first child – which was deeply against my wishes – and so was determined to have a vaginal delivery [or VBAC: vaginal birth after Caesarean section] with my second child. The pregnancy progressed easily, without complications, and I was hoping for a similarly smooth birth. Unfortunately, the shape of my womb meant the baby couldn't rotate properly and so his head couldn't descend. My baby also presented in the occipito-posterior position, which meant I was dilating very slowly and becoming exhausted. The doctors were monitoring me closely but because the baby's heart kept dipping – a possible sign of my Caesarean scar weakening – they were warning that it was likely I would have to have another Caesarean. I was adamant I didn't want it and eventually my second son was born by forceps and ventouse.

When I saw the huge purple bruise over my baby's eye from the forceps, and the bruising on his head from the ventouse, I was overwhelmed with guilt. I felt my need to avoid a Caesarean had been selfish – I had avoided surgery but at a cost to my son who was subsequently born in a forceful way.

Every time I held him in my arms, I couldn't stop kissing his bruises and apologizing for what I had done. I applied arnica cream to the affected areas and he fed ravenously. The bruises faded within two days and I took him to a cranial osteopath a week later. He sent us away without treating the baby, saying there was absolutely no tissue trauma to the head and he was in robust health. His incessant feeding had helped reshape the moulding on his head, but I'm convinced he had accepted my apologies too!

Lack of Help

Another external stress for the depressed mother is insufficient help. Learning about the general care of babies, as well as getting to know your own baby – her character and unique needs – is a full-time job. Keeping the house and providing meals as well is too much for anyone in the immediate post-partum period. It's the antithesis of the red tent concept (see page x) and I strongly advise extra help. Your partner may be off work for the first two weeks but in addition, line up family or very close friends who can help you in the third, fourth and fifth weeks.

Your partner may be off work for the first two weeks but in addition, line up family or very close friends who can help you in the third, fourth and fifth weeks.

Maternity Nurses. You may think of hiring a maternity nurse – a costly but worthwhile investment. The good ones are worth their weight in gold – they can help settle the baby at night after feeds (often the worst part) and help establish a routine – but choose carefully. I strongly recommend choosing from personal recommendations and interviewing before the baby is born.

Night Nannies. Consider a night nanny once or twice a week. They will do the job of the maternity nurse – bringing the baby to you for feeds and settling her afterwards, or just giving a bottle so that you can have an uninterrupted night's sleep – but at a fraction of the cost.

Doulas. Many women are beginning to turn to doulas for help. 'Doula' is a Greek word that means 'handmaiden' so it encapsulates all the aspects of personal care and help. The doula's training is short and is intended to give her an understanding of how to be present as a companion to the mother during birthing. Some doulas are more than birth support partners, but are also trained in therapies that will help the progress of labour. Postnatally, your doula may agree to help with the cooking and housework. Of course, to avoid disappointment you must ask your chosen doula what her role will be both during and after the birth – clarify everything well in advance. I have had feedback that some doulas may decline to help around the house, especially if you already have another young child. In this case it might be better to arrange additional home help.

birth acceptance

Why did I not know that birth is the pinnacle where women discover the courage to be mothers?
The Red Tent

Few of us have fairytale lives, but for most women, life is nonetheless a series of stories with a distinct beginning, middle and end: the wax, plateau and wane of relationships; dating, engagement and marriage; pregnancy, birth and motherhood. All follow a natural life cycle which we neatly précis and shape into stories to share and bond with our friends.

At every NCT (National Childbirth Trust) group across the country, thousands of women who are practically strangers to each other sit drinking tea with babes in arms and recounting their birth stories in explicit detail. This scene is repeated across the world as women forge friendships out of the universality of this uniquely female experience. It's a bonding exercise, but also a catharsis.

Knowing and accepting your birth story is one of the most important elements of embracing motherhood. Before you can become a happy mother, you have to be happy with how you *became* a mother.

Knowing and accepting your birth story is one of the most important elements of embracing motherhood. Before you can become a happy mother, you have to be happy with how you *became* a mother. So many problems can stem from denial of this – postnatal depression, low libido, trouble bonding with the baby, fear of getting pregnant again – and I always urge my mothers to write down their birth experience. Many send their stories in to me, as I of course have a great interest in their pregnancy and birth, and I try to learn something new with the hindsight of each tale.

There are lessons to be learnt even from the archetypal gentle birth. But if you experienced complications during the birth – as so very many mothers do – addressing the issues it throws up is key. Many women feel violated if instrumentation was used; disappointed if they had to have a Caesarean section; or robbed of the entire experience if they delivered under a general anaesthetic. In all events it is good to have a friend or confidant with whom you can talk about your true feelings openly, as sharing your story will make you feel understood.

Of course, for some of you, going over every last detail might be the last thing you want to do, but you will invariably learn something that might alter the course next time. If you can, sit down with your midwife or obstetrician – ideally before you are sent home and the experience is as fresh in their minds – and ask pertinent questions like:

- Was the baby breech because of the shape of my womb?
- Why didn't I dilate quickly?
- Why couldn't the baby turn?
- Was Caesarean really the only option?
- Did the epidural slow down my contractions?

They will know whether your pelvis is shallow or deep, if the baby was too big for your frame or if your vaginal muscles were too tight to avoid an episiotomy. You can't change the past but you can forgive it. By being armed with full knowledge, you can make the changes you need to shape your future – and get your happy ending.

Following is a birth acceptance visualization, which I hope will enable you to experience the kind of positive uplift you can receive as a new mother – whatever your birth story. If you followed the gentle birth method, you will already know how to invoke deep muscle relaxation. To start, sit in a warm, dim place, ideally stretched out in a position you can comfortably maintain for 20 minutes.

Note: If you have a close friend or partner who can read this to you, close your eyes and get into a comfortable position of rest and relaxation, making sure you are warm. Ask them to read very, very slowly and in a soft voice:

Birth Acceptance Visualization

Take three deep breaths into the lowest part of your tummy and let your breath go all the way down into your pelvis. As you breathe out, visualize that your pelvic muscles are utilizing the new oxygen you have just breathed in, and are revitalizing and toning up your amazing birthing spaces. After those three initial breaths, breathe more normally. As you do so, remember that when you close your eyes, you automatically generate the alpha-wave patterns within your brain that induce meditation and a receptive frame of mind!

Take another deep breath to indicate your readiness to let your subconscious send positive messages to your mind and body for total healing, so that you can glorify the fact that you have given birth.

Your soul accepted becoming a mother quite spontaneously and unconsciously, and when you learnt you were pregnant you generously welcomed your tiny little baby into your womb. Your baby grew within your womb for ten whole lunar months, and all the while you talked to your baby and watched your baby grow. You have been so generous with your love!

Of course your baby too gave you untold joy while within your womb, especially when you noticed your friends and even people walking by on the street looking at you with warmth, pride and even curiosity! You pretended to ignore their curiosity but you felt proud within as you smiled to yourself and walked away.

As your baby's birthing day was approaching, you enjoyed curling up on a sofa and tuning in to your thoughts. You visualized holding your baby in your arms and rocking your baby to sleep. The most intimate moments of your baby's life were while you were still carrying your baby within your womb. You intimately shared every thought, every emotion, every rush of love! The closest relationship between two individuals is the relationship of you, the mother, with your baby within your womb. You look back and remember the joy you experienced when your baby moved reassuringly and prodded, nudged and kicked you from within your womb!

Half open your eyes and look around, then close your eyes again as you take three more deep breaths. And as you do so, all your happy moments that you can recall during your pregnancy will flash before your eyes as vivid colourful images – all bright, all beautiful! Almost as if you are seeing yourself in a television screen. Every time you take three deep breaths from now on you will instantly tune in to those wonderful memories that awaken in you feelings of great joy!

You begin to tune in to the fact that the whole purpose of getting pregnant was to hold your tiny baby in your arms and nurture your precious bundle! Your strong maternal instinct is ever-present, even when you are tired, and your baby knows that instinctively. After all, your baby was within your womb all those months and has become finely tuned to the way that you express yourself. You even notice that people on the street smile at you as you walk around your neighbourhood with your baby. They seem to be unconsciously drawn to your subtle radiance.

All that we visualize becomes a reality, so let us visualize that from this moment onwards every time you wish your baby would go to sleep, he/she will … Close your eyes and visualize two special guardian angels spreading their wings of protection around you and your baby, making both of you equally sleepy. Their presence radiates warm waves of sedation that surround you and your baby like a magnetic blanket, sending you both into a wonderful sleep! As you fall into a deep and dreamless sleep, the kind that automatically nurtures and nourishes you and makes you feel immersed in our great universe, you receive an insight that everything you visualize becomes a reality. And you visualize physical help and emotional support for you and your baby for each and every moment of your life.

I invite you to know that each and every birth is unique. You allow your inner mind to forgive your busy lifestyle that might have compromised your birth fitness, and you resolve that next time you will give yourself the total rest that you, as a pregnant mother, truly deserve.

Even though your birth was different from what you expected, we are going to now use your special gift to visualize what your birth should have been like. So let us imagine you and your baby's guardian angel. She is sweeping her arms across the sky as your first contractions come on, sprinkling you in snowflakes which tumble over your hair and down your shoulders, easing all the tension out of your muscles, until your body melts into the consistency of softly set jelly. As you relax, she whispers into the ear of your partner. He envisages his beautiful baby inside your body, preparing to be born, dropping down all the way into your pelvis with the baby's chin on his/her chest so that his/her head is well flexed and fits easily into your inner pelvic space, ready to smoothly slide down your birthing spaces ... stretching and moulding all the way down to your vaginal opening. You visualize your baby actively participating in the birth process by secreting even more elastin and relaxin that automatically widen and soften your pelvic spaces, magically expanding them into a wide-open channel for your birth process.

From where we are now, your angel eases the tenderness and the tissue memory from all of your muscles that are healing so well. Your angel understands and transmits to your inner mind what you needed to know at the time of your birth so that you forgive the past easily and proceed to heal smoothly.

Your inner mind suddenly becomes aware that both you and your baby have together created a wide-open channel within your pelvis that a tiny baby can easily slide out of. Check this out with your inner mind, and if your inner mind agrees then take a deep breath in and out and let your whole body relax even further as you allow all the tissues in your body to behave as if they have just experienced your dream birth!

Take another deep breath in and out as you ask all the tissues in your body, especially in your pelvis and birthing areas, to release all old tissue memories and imprint the new visualized memory of the birth that you and your baby have now created within your minds.

Take another deep breath into the lowest part of your tummy and ask your amazing inner mind to let your eyes open ... only ... when your inner mind has totally integrated this special healing into all the parts of your mind and into your tissue memory.

questions to ask after an assisted delivery

Following an instrumented delivery, such as a ventouse birth, you may want to ask your doctor or midwife the following questions to get a better idea of what was needed and why, its effect on the baby, and whether it'll be necessary next time.

1 Was the baby's head fairly well down or was it quite high in the pelvis?
2 Was the suction pressure increased too quickly?
3 Was the traction applied forceful or gentle?
4 Was the baby's head delivered slowly and gently?
5 Was it wise to attempt a vaginal delivery i.e. if the baby was too big to fit through the mother's pelvis?
6 What was the condition of the maternal tissues – swollen or rigid?

A careful and skilful obstetrician can indeed minimize the risks to mother and baby. As always, prevention is better than cure. I advocate that all mothers try and follow the guidelines set out in my first book, *The Gentle Birth Method*, so that even in the eventuality of an instrumental delivery there can be easier application of the instruments with a gentler delivery for the baby.

A good homeopathic remedy to help ease the disappointment of instrumentation or a Caesarean section is staphysagria 200c immediately after the birth and, if possible, three times a day for three days afterwards.

baby
post-partum care

Here is a summary of useful treatments and care techniques for the baby in the first week after birth.

Light reflexology. At this point, it's more of a gentle foot massage for the baby. Very gently lift your baby's foot and softly massage the toes, one by one. Then, with either the heel of your hand or the knuckle of your crooked index finger, lightly stroke the soles of the feet in an upward direction. This area helps digestion and encourages the baby to relax, and it's something you can do easily whilst feeding.

Cupping and cooling. Otherwise known as 'stroking the aura', this non-touch remedy can really soothe irritable babies. Put a drop of Rescue Remedy onto some cotton wool and wipe it over the fontanelles. Then mould your hand into a cup shape and, at a distance of one inch from the baby's head, gently make long sweeping strokes in one direction only, from the baby's forehead to the occiput at the back of her head. Repeat for at least five minutes, and up to twenty minutes, as often as you like daily.

Cranio-sacral therapy. Take the baby to a reputed practitioner in the first few days after the birth, especially if your labour was long or instrumentation was used. Go, too, if you had a Caesarean. A good cranial practitioner can make a big difference if your baby is fractious, irritable, difficult to settle, or suffered moulding to the head during the birth.

Cleaning the umbilical stump. Do this twice a day with a solution of 20ml of boiled and cooled water, mixed with a drop of tea tree oil.

Eye contact. Make lots of eye contact with your baby, especially when talking to her. You may well find your voice is naturally higher and softer than normal. This is known as 'motherese' and is an instinctive response – babies find it easier to listen to a higher-pitched voice.

Holding your baby. Your newborn baby feels most secure and is easiest to hold when snugly wrapped in the swaddling blanket and held up with her head nuzzling into your neck. There's a natural nook for her there, and she can rest her head and smell your hair. Baby bliss.

Sleep. Place your baby to sleep in a small space, such as a Moses basket, *thottil*, hammock or crib. Avoid letting her sleep in the car seat as lying in this crouched position for too long can cause her blood circulation to pool. Allow your baby to sleep as long as she wants to between feeds.

Swaddling. During naps, fully swaddle the baby to make her feel secure and held (see box), and to minimize the Moro reflex.

Nappy changes. Keep them brief – dress the baby in sleep suits with leg and crotch poppers to minimize tugging and wrestling with arms and legs. This will cut down on crying time in the first days.

Songs and Lullabies. Choose a short song or lullaby that you would like to sing to your baby every day. Sing it whenever you do a nappy change, or softly hum it during feeds. Let her associate the tune with closeness and care from you.

Winding. This should be gentle and relaxed. Many mothers frantically jiggle their babies on their knees, or pat their back hard, or rock them backwards and forwards to encourage the burps to come up. I have always felt that the gentler the touch, the more relaxed the baby will be – and if she's relaxed, there'll be less resistance or internal tension keeping the wind down. Only wind when the baby has naturally broken off during the feed, and again at the end of the feed. Gently sit the baby up and, holding her under the arms, lift her just off your knees so that she is stretched out and her body is stretched long under her full weight. Hold for a moment, then return her to a sitting position on your lap. Place her chin in the cradle of your hand (between thumb and index finger) and put your other hand on her back. Gently stroke the back rhythmically, preferably only in a downward direction. Pause frequently to 'allow' the baby to bring up the wind. Another winding method is to rest her on your shoulder with her arms hanging over your shoulder and down your back (the positioning is crucial for this method). This places light pressure on her abdomen, and the stretched-out position makes it easier for the air bubbles to come up. Place a cloth over your shoulder to protect your clothes!

mother
birth recovery

Arnica. Take immediately after the birth and then every thirty minutes for the first five days. Arnica is very important in reducing post-partum bruising and swelling, even after the gentlest birth.

Hypericum. If you had a Caesarean or suffered a tear/episiotomy, take 200c immediately after the birth and every six hours for five days.

Painkillers. Take as necessary if prescribed by the hospital if you have had a Caesarean or an episiotomy.

Ice packs. If your perineum feels bruised and sore after a vaginal birth you could apply an ice pack for ten minutes, three times a day, whilst sitting or lying down. You can bathe your perineum with cotton swabs soaked in a solution of 50ml of water containing ten to twenty drops of the mother tincture of calendula.

Supplements. Start taking vitamin B_{12} and Floradix (a natural iron supplement) to help build up your haemoglobin levels. This will counteract the effects of any significant blood loss during the birth. Anaemia can cause tiredness, anxiety and dizzy spells. Take 500mg vitamin C daily. This is important for the cell membranes and will speed healing in all your tissues after birth.

Massage. In India, it is traditional to massage the mother from the day of the birth using Ayurvedic oils. As is the custom, the pregnant mother goes to live with her mother and gives birth in her childhood home. Then her mother or aunt will massage her daily with warm coconut or cured sesame oil. The more aware women use Ayurvedic oils. I adapt this for Western cultures by advocating a rose otto oil massage (see page

46). This will help lift your mood and banish the baby blues. Repeat daily if possible.

Ayurvedic herbs. Baladi choornam tones up the uterus as it involutes (the same herb I prescribe in my first book, *The Gentle Birth Method*). It is also a strengthening herb. Take once a day after your evening meal for a total of forty days postnatally (see Resources for details). The following Ayurvedic elixirs taste like sweet sherry:

- Jeerarishtam helps to bring in your milk: the main ingredient is cumin. (See recipe on page 38 for substitute fennel tonic.)
- Dashamoolarishtam tightens the pelvic ligaments and tones the uterus.
- Dhanwantaram kashayam tastes like bitters and is also prescribed for postnatal recovery of the tissues.

Visualizations. From the first day, practise daily, short visualizations of your uterus involuting and shrinking back into the pelvis – imagine it becoming small, round and tight, like a tennis ball. You may well feel afterpains. This is due to the fact that suckling stimulates the release of oxytocin, the hormone responsible for the womb contracting. This helps your uterus involute and return to its pre-pregnant size. So please practise these visualizations during feed times and whenever you have a moment when you can sit down, close your eyes and relax!

Take a shower. Preferably take a shower in the hospital. If you have been sent home within the first twenty-four hours, then you could have a shower or short bath at home. Beware: too hot a bath may cause you to have heavier lochia (vaginal bleeding). There is always some degree of bruising in the vagina, so avoid prolonged baths within the first twenty-four hours as bruised tissue is more susceptible to absorbing water, swelling up and getting infected.

Healing waters. After day two, run a bath of warm water (about 36 degrees centigrade) and add a herbal infusion made up of dried marjoram flowers, comfrey leaves and St John's wort leaves and flowers (see Resources for stockists). Wrap up a handful of each of these three herbs in a muslin cloth and let this bundle steep in a litre of boiling water for twenty minutes. Then decant and pour into your normal bath water. It smells bitter and looks dark brown, but it will relax you profoundly, ease all your muscles and heal your perineum really quickly. If you prefer, you can infuse some camomile tea bags in a teapot and pour the lot – including the teabags – into the bath. Birth utilizes a lot of nervous energy, and camomile is renowned for its soothing effect on the nervous system. It is also very good for repairing damaged local tissues.

Drink two litres of water a day. This will encourage milk production.

Add lemon or cranberry juice to your drinking water. This will alkalinize your urine, helping to prevent cystitis, which is very common in the first few days after birth.

Toilet trips. You will find you are going to the toilet a lot. This is because your body is shedding up to five litres of extra fluid from your blood volume that was required during the pregnancy.

Light reflexology. From day one, ask your partner to massage your feet, working especially on the tops of the feet where the tendons are. This pertains to the breast reflexes and encourages good milk let-down.

Take Lactors. This is a homeopathic remedy I source from a 96-year-old homeopath in India. It helps create better quality milk that can calm irritable babies. Available to order from our website www.gentlebirthmethod.com (see Resources for details).

Feeding. Feed yourself and your baby on demand!

Diet. Be vigilant in following a low-fibre diet but with the addition of gentle greens like steamed runner beans and okra for the first few weeks, to protect from constipation. The strain of pushing when constipated can cause pressure on fresh episiotomy or Caesarean scars. Prunes and figs and cooked beetroot can really help in loosening your bowels to help you eliminate easily. You may have been prescribed lactulose by your doctor but this can only do so much – make diet your main priority. Remember the fish soup for non-vegetarians and other calcium-rich foods. For both vegetarians and non-vegetarians, pear compote and my favourite postnatal pudding, *kullie*, provide additional sources of natural calcium (see recipe on page 35).

- Foods to include: plums, compote, figs, prunes, porridge, soft soups (particularly organic chicken soup), asparagus, butternut squash, all legumes
- Foods to avoid – brassica family (wind-producing), such as cabbage, cauliflowers, Brussels sprouts; also refrain from eating tomatoes, citrus fruits and grapes.

Opening your bowels. When you have to open your bowels, place a clean sanitary pad either against your Caesarean scar or episiotomy on the perineum, and very gently apply external support to the wound. Relax and let natural peristalsis expel the waste.

Haemorrhoids. These are a common postnatal symptom. Here is a useful tip contributed by one of my mothers: soak a round cotton wool pad in some witch hazel and tuck into the crack between your buttocks so that it lies against the haemorrhoids; this astringent causes the swelling to subside. (See also page 284.)

Eat protein. Protein in the breastfeeding mother's diet has been shown to have a calming effect on the baby.

Probiotic supplements. If you have been taking probiotics and digestive enzymes during your pregnancy, please continue taking them or start taking them now as they will optimize your digestive health and improve the quality of your milk, reducing fretfulness in the baby. My favourite is by the brand MORDHA, which provides a capsule-a-day dose of concentrated filtered fish oil, specially recommended for pregnant and lactating mothers. This also acts as an antidepressant. If you are breastfeeding, it goes through to your baby and helps brain development (see Resources).

---

ideal eating plan for the first few days

Breakfast: Porridge with chopped banana, raisins, nuts and maple syrup *or* stewed fruit and honey. Ideally, drink water one to two hours after solid food so that your digestive juices can mix with the food in a high concentration (drinking too much water with food dilutes your digestive juices, interfering with thorough digestion and leading to bloating).

Mid-morning snack: Serve yoghurt or fruit separately.

Lunch: Sardines on (preferably wheat-free) toast, lemon and ginger tea *or* steamed vegetables *or* chicken breast and salad or fish soup.

Supper: Full English roast (preferably organic chicken) or Thai green chicken curry made with coconut milk (minimal curry paste and lashings of vegetables). For vegetarians, kitchidi served with vegetable curry or stew. Suitable hot drinks include ginger, camomile or fennel tea.

---

by day five

By day five or so, see a creative healing practitioner or ask your partner to perform a female treatment (see Resources for a do-at-home DVD). This incorporates:

Pelvic lift: The weight of the pregnant uterus places pressure on the ligaments and needs to be lifted back up after birth; it also redirects the energy lines back to the uterus.

Pelvic drainage: Clearing away the excess fluids and congestion in the pelvic cavity.

Abdominal toning: Encouraging the abdominal muscles to sit back together and helping tone the stretched skin.

Heart treatment: The heart hypertrophies (enlarges) by thirty per cent during pregnancy to cope with the extra circulatory load, and also works very hard during birth. Like your uterus, your heart also has to go back to its pre-pregnant shape, size and tone. A creative healing heart treatment can be useful.

Bladder drainage: Along with pelvic drainage, this drains the lymphatics of the bladder and can prevent cystitis, a common postnatal condition. Often the urethra gets bruised or compressed during birth, and creative healing drainage can reduce fluid retention in that area and assist healing.

MOXIBUXTION TECHNIQUE

Sonia Revelli, one of my gentle birth mothers, swears by a practice called mother roasting! This is done on day five after the birth to energize the mother and aid her recovery. A moxa stick is burned and the hot tip waved above the mother's abdomen (travelling up and down the midline of the abdomen from the acupuncture point Ren 2 to Ren 8 and back again) for five to ten minutes. (The acupressure points Du 2 and Du 4 can also be warmed.) If the mother has a fever or night sweats then please refrain from performing this moxibuxtion.

BOOST YOUR MILK SUPPLY

If your milk supply needs a boost, drink fennel tonic, which can also help prevent colic in the baby (see recipe on page 38). Alternatively, make an infusion by adding the following herbs to one pint of very hot water:

1 teaspoon each of

dried raspberry leaves
dried nettle leaves
rosehips
burdock root
dried camomile flowers
fennel seeds
dried alfa-alfa leaves (if you can find it)

Allow the mixture to steep for twenty minutes, then strain and drink.

CATNAP

Catnap as often as you can. If you have followed the gentle birth method, you will be able to use your capacity to day-dream, lead yourself into a self-hypnotic sleep and easily drift off into a deep sleep. You can preset the number of minutes that you want to sleep for, and you will be surprised how your eyes will open automatically after that set length of time!

STAY AT HOME!

Rest … and put off all non-essential visitors in the first week. Your baby has just arrived in a new environment and you are gently introducing her to new substances within your home so that she can develop antibodies in stages. Limiting visitors avoids overloading your baby's immune system. Of course, after a few weeks your baby will be more immune competent and thus able to cope with more antigens and the general public!

LIMIT YOUR PHONE CALLS

Lastly, please avoid phone calls while you are breastfeeding. Your baby does benefit from your undivided attention at these precious moments. Avoid using your mobile phone around your baby. I am very concerned about the long-term effects of microwaves on your brain and on your baby's immune system.

birth-specific treatments for mother and baby
episiotomy, vaginal bruising, ventouse

mother

- To reduce bruising and swelling, take arnica 30c every fifteen to thirty minutes immediately after the birth for a couple of hours and then six-hourly for five days.
- To make a healing solution, mix ten drops of the mother tincture of hypericum with half a cup of water. Use the solution to bathe the tissues in the area that needs healing. This is suitable for all degrees of bruising, cuts or tears. Even after a normal birth, mothers have to heal their vaginal muscles, which undergo great expansion to deliver the baby.
- Use an ice pack to soothe and reduce swelling in the perineal area. Apply to the affected area for ten to fifteen minutes, perhaps three times a day.
- To help mothers emotionally accept the fact that instrumentation was necessary, take staphisagria 200c three times a day for five days.
- To soften the stools and prevent constipation, relieving pressure on the healing tissues, take lactulose – 10 to 15ml a day, three times a day for three days. Of course I am a great believer in creative healing to relieve constipation (see Resources).
- To help you relax and feel sedated, have a camomile tea bath. This can also have a soothing effect on your muscles. Take six camomile tea bags, place in a litre of boiling water in a saucepan for fifteen minutes then simmer for ten minutes. Allow this to cool and add the infusion to a warm bath at 34 degrees centigrade.
- After six weeks, your doctor, midwife or a highly skilled cranial osteopath can apply a fascial unwind to your vaginal tissues. This will thin and loosen the vaginal or abdominal scar tissue. Even mothers who have had normal vaginal births could suffer internal bruising that goes unnoticed until sexual activity is resumed.

- Impressive healing can be obtained by using our minds, so visualize the tissues knitting together completely within a few days. And you will be surprised how quickly you heal.
- During labour, your baby's head may have been pressing down on your bladder neck and part of your bladder wall. This pressure could cause oedema (fluid retention) and make you prone to cystitis. You can drain and cool the delicate tissues within your bladder by applying a daily creative healing cooling treatment to the lower abdomen for three days, along with pelvic drainage massage (see at-home DVD, Resources). Along with this please drink plenty of water with a squeeze of lemon. Lemon and cranberry juices are invaluable for alkalinizing your urine, thereby preventing cystitis.

caesarean birth

mother

- To prevent bruising and swelling, take hypericum 200c every six hours for the first three days.
- Refrain from baths for at least seven days after the Caesarean section as the area where your skin was sutured should be dry. This is more of a cosmetic consideration. In theory, the skin actually knits together within twenty-four hours but it does take at least seven days for the scar to organize and seal off the subcutaneous tissue.
- Take lactulose to prevent constipation. Straining may exert painful pressure on the healing wound and cause pain.
- If there was a pushing phase during birth, the stress on the rectal wall may have caused haemorrhoids (see witch hazel tip on page 63). There is also a very efficient treatment for haemorrhoids in creative healing (see resources for do-at-home DVD).
- To help you come to terms with an operative birth, take staphisagria 30c three times a day for five days.

- To help your milk come in – usually delayed by a couple of days for Caesarean-section mothers – I recommend my favourite remedy Lactors (see Resources for stockist).
- Vitamin B_{12} is always a useful supplement as it is essential for the stability of the central nervous system, can prevent postnatal depression and is also useful for recovery of cut or damaged nerves.
- Iron supplements are generally a good idea as there is usually a greater blood loss during Caesarean section. Ideally, opt for the more natural bio-absorbable form of iron supplementation like Floradex, and iron-rich foods.

---

cosmetic tip

To reduce scar tissue formation after a Caesarean section, it may be a good idea to wear a compression bandage over the lower abdomen. This is a special pressure garment. A plastic surgeon can measure you and order one for you. You will then have to wear it almost all the time for at least six months to one year. This has an amazing effect and your scar will hardly be noticeable. I would certainly recommend this measure if you have noticed an increased keloid scar tendency on other areas of your body where you have had a cut or a bruise. In general, keloid scars can be rather itchy and painful. If you already have a keloid scar, you could have it surgically revised by a sensitive plastic surgeon but the post-operative care with the pressure garment is vitally important.

baby

CRANIO-SACRAL THERAPY

This seems to be gaining popularity and acceptance in the neonatal world. The birth process, even when natural, can impose certain stresses and strains on the baby's cranium, and the professional cranio-sacral therapist will ascertain these stresses and help to unwind these patterns. Even in the gentlest of births the fact that the baby was head-down in the mother's womb prior to birth would have led to more compression on one side of the cranium. As a mother, you may notice that your baby favours turning her neck to one side, which is mostly due to pre-birth positioning within the womb.

WATER THERAPY

The simplest therapy for you and your baby would be to get into a bath at 36 degrees centigrade. Then support your baby lightly in the bath with your hands, floating her on her back first facing you and then facing away from you as you place one hand under the baby's bottom. With your other hand, cup your baby's cranium, making sure the whole of your baby's chin and face floats above the level of water. You will notice your baby naturally move from side to side as you follow with your hands, and then your baby will try to twist her trunk in a way that suggests fascial unwinding. This is a great, gentle form of do-it-yourself fascial unwind for the baby.

* Fascia is connective tissue that may store tension left over from the positions in the womb or obtained from the birth process. If left unwound, fascial tissues can restrict the way muscles move in childhood. These patterns might persist into adulthood. By helping the baby unwind, you assist normal infant growth and development.

--- **tip for defying gravity** -------------------------------

Spending time in the water also counteracts the effects of gravity. Most of our oxygen consumption goes to counteract the effect of gravity. Hence your baby will be able to utilize the greater circulating levels of oxygen for brain growth and development. And you will also be able to benefit from the extra oxygen to revive those tired brain cells!

CUPPING AND COOLING

This creative healing method can help to reverse the moulding of the head that can occur at birth. There is an energy field all around us. In babies, whose tissues are delicate, the energy fields are more open and easily helped. The simplest form of therapy is to cup the aura or energy field around your baby's head by scooping the air above the head in a one-directional cooling movement with the intention of restoring the tissues to greater comfort levels. I like to start at the eyebrows and stroke over and above the head towards the base of the cranium at the top of the neck. This is also called the 'cooling breeze'. Anyone can do this safely and it is marvellous immediately after the birth! It seems to take away internal heat and inflammation that could be caused by the birth, especially if the pushing phase was long. You will notice the immediate effects of your cupping and cooling movements, as your baby will look really relaxed and will fall into a deep sleep.

pre-term babies

- You might find the baby's head so tiny that you wonder how to comfort her. Apply the cupping treatment over your baby's head as described above. This will be invaluable in helping to stabilize all of your baby's brain membranes and cranial blood vessels, making her feel safe and calm.

- Reiki is a gentle, non-invasive, light form of touch or off-the-body healing that can be given to your baby.
- Kangaroo mother care (see page 22) – breastfeed your baby (express your milk until such time as you can directly feed the baby); hold, cuddle and massage your baby as much as possible. Go skin-to-skin at every opportunity – the mother's body contact and light touch has the ultimate healing power.

two to twelve weeks

baby

crying

crying as communication

There are few things harder for the new mother to bear than the sound of her baby crying. She can cope with the broken nights, hours of breastfeeding and four to six weeks of postnatal lochia (bleeding), but one wail from her baby can bring everything to a halt until she has discovered the cause of her baby's unhappiness. And there's the rub. Because where adults cry from sadness or pain (and the occasional soppy film), babies use crying as a means of bringing attention to the fact they are cold, hot, hungry, windy, bored, tired, overtired, sitting in a dirty nappy, lying in a wet vest … In other words, anything at all.

Where adults cry from sadness or pain, babies use crying as a means of bringing attention to the fact they are cold, hot, hungry, windy, bored, tired, overtired, sitting in a dirty nappy, lying in a wet vest … anything at all.

If babies were born with the power of speech, the vast majority of new mothers would find motherhood a breeze. Just imagine: 'Did you say you're cold, darling? Let's put on your cardigan.' 'Sorry, what's that? You're bored of sitting under your gym? Let's go for a walk.' 'Is that really the time? – no wonder you're hungry.' Caring for a newborn isn't brain surgery – it's just like trying to look after someone who only speaks ancient Greek. Frustrating, baffling and long-winded.

Once you accept that your baby crying doesn't mean he is sad or in pain (although of course, sometimes it may) and he is simply asking you to remedy a frustration or minor situation, your anxiety levels will drop dramatically and your confidence will grow. But in the beginning, this heightened state of alert is completely understandable. Your body is hormonally programmed to respond to your baby's cries – your heart rate will quicken, you'll have a burst of adrenaline, and your milk will be let down. It's an evolutionary response which is overridden only by the confidence that comes with experience, and eventually you'll know what he wants even before you've picked him up. Initially, your baby's cries will sound indistinct to you, but your ear will rapidly become trained to the small nuances which distinguish one from another.

types of crying

Pain	High pitched, loud, incessant; will make you instinctively run.
Tired	Reaches crescendo and tails off into mewing; regular pauses, increasing in length and frequency.
Lonely/bored	Quieter, growing in volume; regular pauses.
Discomfort	Irregular cries accompanied by wriggling.
Hunger	Rhythmic, often accompanied by kicking out.

The most important thing is to respond to your baby's cry quickly. Even if you can't work out immediately what is wrong, just by holding and soothing your baby, he will be calmed to some degree until you discover the root cause. This checklist usually eliminates most causes:

Even if after eight weeks the cries still all sound the same to you, take heart. Around this age, your baby will begin to cry less as he discovers other ways to communicate his needs to you. Facilitate this by making lots of eye contact, especially when you are speaking to your baby. Point to objects and name them for your baby, and explain what you're doing as you go about your day together: 'Now I'm going to put you in the pram…' The more you inform your baby of his world, the more quickly he will join it, and the less either of you will have to cope with crying as communication.

COLIC

Of course, if your baby is crying incessantly, this is not normal and should be investigated for any underlying medical reason. Reflux is a consideration (see page 265) but colic is the most common diagnosis, usually coming on by three weeks, peaking at six and abating by twelve weeks. Often it is worst during the early evening period (5–8pm) but it can strike more randomly and is usually defined as three hours of crying, at least three days a week, for at least three weeks. If you suspect colic, try the following precautions:

- Perform the Ayurvedic baby leg stretches (see page 19) at each nappy change.
- Visit a reputed cranio-sacral therapist as soon as possible. Magical results can be had from a cranial session. Often intra-cranial stresses and strains can lead to a crying infant. A series of cranial treatments can decompress and restore cranial rhythms, and calm your baby down. A good cranial practitioner can ease your baby's discomfort in a couple of sessions.
- Give a drop of Infacol before each feed to facilitate winding. This will help form bigger bubbles in the tummy, making it easier to burp the baby.
- Alternatively, offer a teaspoon of gripe water after each feed. The main ingredient in gripe water is fennel seeds.
- When the baby breaks off from the breast naturally during a feed, sit him up and do some gentle winding by alternately tapping the back gently with the palm of one hand and stroking the back in a downward manner. Once you hear a satisfactory burp, resume the feed.
- Make sure the baby has finished on the first breast before offering the second.
- Consult a homeopath for a good constitutional remedy for you and your baby.
- Keep your diet as close to your antenatal diet as possible.
- Eliminate from your diet caffeine, alcohol and wind-producing foods such as sprouts, cabbage, broccoli and beans.
- Drink nettle or fennel tea. Steep one teaspoon in half a pint of hot water for ten minutes. Then strain and drink.
- Try some gentle baby massage before the usual crying period.
- Hold your baby in the Tiger in the Tree position to minimize crying. Lay the baby face-down on your forearm with your palm face up. Let your baby's arms and legs hang on either side of your forearm. The baby's head should nestle and be supported in the crook of your arm. Stroke and pat the baby's back gently.

two to twelve weeks

- Keep close at all times. My favourite cure is a form of purring lullaby where I make an 'rrrrrrrrr' sound by lightly placing the tip of my tongue on the front of my hard palate and hum a tune making 'rrrrrrrrr' sounds that catch the baby's attention. You can even hum a whole tune like the Brahms *Lullaby* to the 'rrrrrrrrr' sound!
- Sing your special song over and over again to calm and relax yourself and your baby.
- I have often found it equally important to treat the mother as it is to treat the baby. A series of reflexology or cranial treatments for the mother have proved to be lifesavers. A good homeopath can prescribe some remedies that can really help to calm your fears and balance your hormones. Remember that the baby can pick up the mother's unconscious fears and anxieties and reflect them by being unsettled. A calm mother equals a calm baby.

crying and survival Instinct

In evolutionary terms, your baby's survival depends upon bonding with you. In the beginning, crying is his only way of communicating with you. He'll scream to be fed immediately because food is the first primal need for your baby. Hunger could be a new sensation for your baby as in the womb he was drip-fed by the placenta. But babies are also intuitive and quickly learn that their survival depends upon getting your attention and winning your love. Your baby soon sees how to elicit your delight with a smile! Slowly, positive communication replaces crying as the dialogue between you improves. Rest assured that however well you may think you know your baby, your baby knows you better!

sleep

overtiredness

Crying is also a problem when the baby is tired or trying to go to sleep. Sleep is a natural instinct but also a skill that has to be learnt – something easier said than done.

Sleep is as crucial to babies as milk in the early months – it's when they grow and the brain hard-wires daily routine into experience – so it is your responsibility to make sure they get enough of it.

Head shaking, pulling away, eye rubbing, staring into the distance and kicking out with the legs are all signs of tiredness, and once you tip over into overtiredness (even by ten minutes), it will be harder to settle the baby to sleep. Watch the clock and start to observe the baby's behaviour after an hour of being up and about. If he is showing any of the above signs, swaddle him and soothe him with a cuddle and song, or gently stroke his head to wind him down. Slowing your breathing and taking long, deep breaths will encourage him to reset his breathing pattern naturally. After a few minutes of this he should be happy to be placed in his cot with the mechanical musical mobile on. A few minutes' crying whilst he 'settles' is normal but that should soon turn into a 'mewing', which means sleep is coming on.

If the baby has already tipped over into overtiredness and has launched into a crying spasm, watch over him without picking him up. Stroke his forehead, do some cupping to 'stroke his aura' (see page 21), or just lay a comforting hand on his tummy. Trust in his natural ability to fall asleep. Turn on his mobile and make sure there is some soft music playing to comfort him– even if he is determined to drown it out!

If he persists in crying then pick him up and gently sway him in your arms (not jigging or bouncing). I swear by figure-of-eight hip and shoulder swivels. Use the dummy if need be until he is fully pacified and calmed down, then gently put him down and try again. It's much harder getting an overtired baby off to sleep, and if picking up and soothing three or four times over a period of forty-five minutes to one hour doesn't work, then abandon the sleep period and focus on something else, such as going for a walk. It's guaranteed that he'll nod off within moments in the pram/sling/car/baby swing as most babies cannot stay awake with motion in the first month.

---

tip: rousing baby from sleeping on the breast

Sleeping on the breast is especially difficult to prevent in the early days when the delightful feeling of a warm, milky tummy is too much for a little baby to resist. All they want is to sleep at the source of this ambrosia. It's lovely for the mother too, but ultimately it doesn't encourage good feeding or sleeping habits, so a little tickle on the soles of the feet can rouse the baby just long enough for him to be aware of being placed in his cot. If you want to wake the baby to continue with the feed, raise his arm like a lever. It's gentle but effective.

getting your baby to sleep

Many experts warn against certain measures to get the baby to sleep – such as rocking, patting, using a dummy or feeding – but I understand how hard this can be. It's our instinct to console a crying baby by these methods, and I think it's fine to use them for the first few weeks if you feel you need to. Just try to use them at a minimal level and keep in mind that any shortcut habits created now will only have to be broken later – it's usually a matter of when, not if.

I do recommend you put your baby to sleep in the cot, rather than out in the pram or in the car. For one thing, a better quality of sleep will be enjoyed in the cot. If, however, your baby needs motion to settle down to sleep, then that means you're the one having to move about. Keep in mind the red tent concept that you rest *together*. You could use your baby's naps as your own rest periods too. You will be so thankful for that quiet, still time to yourself once you have established a sleep routine both of you can trust.

If your baby is crying a bit at bedtime, remember that crying is his only means of communication, and if his tummy is full, he has been winded and his nappy changed, then what you're most likely dealing with is crossness and a little confusion. But if you are persistent, it really only takes most babies a week or two to learn that the answer lies in closing their eyes. Still, until that Eureka moment, many mothers find themselves sitting on the stairs in despair, crying too – it's almost a rite of passage!

Keep your resolve and persist. A rested child is a happier child (and a rested mummy is a better mummy). Your baby will play better and learn more by day, and sleep better and grow more by night.

- All babies love to go to sleep under a musical mobile. Choose one that operates from a silent push-button where the music plays for fifteen minutes, rather than three minutes. Wind-up mechanisms can be ratchety and incredibly noisy and tend to actually wake the baby up, just when he is dropping off to sleep (see Resources for details).
- Have a sleep-time mantra and always say exactly the same thing to the baby when you put him down and leave him – even if you have to go in fifteen times.
- The room should be dim to dark.
- The baby's room temperature should be kept within the recommended band of 16 to 20 degrees centigrade in the winter. In the summer you need to keep the room as cool as possible. If it's very hot and your baby is in a sleeping bag, remember to move down to a 1 tog or 0.5 tog.
- Make sure the baby's room is quieter than the main living areas of the house.
- Any time other than high summer, make sure their feet are covered as their little extremities could get cold and wake them up.
- A cloth book with white/black/red/yellow combinations that can be placed within the cot will provide a distraction and they'll soon learn to anticipate sleep when they are placed next to it.
- One or two (no more) small familiar toys will become comforters, especially if you sleep with them for a couple of days so that they smell of you. (Important note: the toys must be small enough so that they will still be safe in case the baby pulls them over his face.)
- Be consistent and re-create the sleeping environment wherever you are. Even if you travel, take the mobile, toys and cot book with you.
- Sing the same lullaby or tune to your baby as you put him to sleep. If somebody is baby-sitting for you, please make sure that they also sing your sleep-time tune or favourite nursery rhyme that can act as a mantra!

- If your baby was born in the spring then you have the advantage of the warmer summer months to help you. You could hang a wooden wind chime at an open window (the metal ones can be a little tinny to small ears). The soft, low, 'glock' sounds are intrinsically soothing on the breeze and conducive to sleep.

The quicker the baby *associates* these rituals with sleep, the sooner they will automatically *trigger* sleep.

---

seasonal sleep tips

summer babies

It's dreamy for a baby to sleep outdoors, when the temperature permits. Sleeping under a blossom or willow tree is glorious at three weeks, so take every opportunity to indulge your baby. Just make sure you cover the pram with a mosquito or cat net, position the baby out of direct sunlight and make sure he has sufficient covers to counteract any cooling breeze.

winter babies

Try placing your baby to sleep on a baby sheepskin. The sheep blankets made for babies are specially sheared to a shorter length, and are machine washable. They are particularly cosy for winter babies but are also cool in the summer months. You can lay the baby directly on top of the fleece, which is wonderfully comforting, or if you prefer, layer the fleece beneath the cot sheet to provide a soft, insulating base.

When settling a distressed or overtired baby, cradle him in your arms with his head on your left-hand side, next to your heart. Begin to take slower, deeper breaths to mimic the breathing change when asleep. It may take a few minutes but your baby will become attuned to this and begin to relax. Your baby will recognize the slower, deeper breathing pattern and respond in kind.

cot death

This fear surrounding cot death is understandable as the specific causes for it are as yet unknown. Until scientists can pinpoint the exact reasons it occurs, it appears to us to strike at random. However, a process of elimination is gradually identifying avoidable risk factors.

From a medical point of view, we know that cot death is most common in Caucasian babies aged between one and six months, although it can claim children up to eighteen months. (It is very rare in Asian families, possibly because of co-sleeping.) It prevails in conditions where one or both of the parents smoke (including during pregnancy); rooms are overheated or stuffy without good circulation; and where the baby is put to sleep on the tummy or side. On a socio-economic scale it is more common in lower-income families. Since the government set up its awareness campaign in 1991, the incidence of cot deaths has dropped by seventy-five per cent.

precautions to prevent cot death

- If you are swaddling, only ever use a cotton cellular blanket to allow temperature regulation.
- Put baby to sleep on his back.
- Avoid cot bumpers – there is a fear that cot bumpers restrict fresh air circulating around the baby's head.
- Ban smoking around your child, in the baby's room or in your house. There is now very strong evidence that passive smoking directly affects babies. If your baby is invited to sleep in a room where the owners are smokers, get a baby-sitter instead!
- Make sure the room is at the ideal temperature of 16 to 20 degrees centigrade.
- If the baby is sleeping in blankets, make sure his feet are placed at the foot of the cot, so that he can't wriggle down and under the covers. This is known as 'feet to foot'.
- I personally recommend putting your baby to sleep in a sleeping bag (after three weeks of age) as this avoids the risk of the baby's face being covered with the blankets.

In India, we routinely sprinkle frankincense resin powder onto hot embers, and the fragrant incense that rises from the holder is waved underneath the baby's sleeping place every morning and night to purify this precious space. The common understanding is that frankincense clears the air of negative vibrations. If you are religious or spiritual at all, you might like to sprinkle holy water around your baby's cot. Certainly many mothers I know say special little prayers when putting their children to bed and when they go to bed themselves, even if they had never previously considered themselves religious.

massage

One of my favourite Indian baby tips is the warm oil massage. Coconut oil is poured over a whole betel leaf, which is held in the palm of your hand and warmed over hot embers until the leaf is soft and green. The baby is then held over your other forearm and his back, neck, limbs and then tummy are gently stroked and massaged with the warmed betel leaf for fifteen to twenty minutes. The oil is not washed off but left on as a moisturizer. The warmth of the oil and the gentle massage has a sedating effect on the baby. This warm massage with the medicinal leaf and oil was thought to be very important in the tropics for preventing chest infections in babies. Betel leaf also contains certain ingredients that help digestion.

As well as being deeply relaxing for the baby, massage is also an invaluable part of the bonding process and something I strongly recommend to all my mothers (albeit in a modified form – betel leaves aren't quite so readily available on the high street, though they are easily found in Asian shops in the UK). Try sweet almond oil or extra virgin olive oil instead.

Baby massage not only creates a pathway of non-verbal loving dialogue between mother and baby, which makes the baby feel valued and adored, but also boasts many physiological and health benefits, which can't be ignored.

---

health benefits of regular baby massage

- Improves blood circulation.
- Helps with digestion and the release of wind! Especially if you incorporate the Ayurvedic leg stretches into your baby massage routine (see page 19).
- Improves muscle tone.
- Keeps the joints flexible.
- Promotes growth by stimulating the pituitary gland to release growth hormone.
- Boosts immunity as lymphocytes migrate to the surface of the skin wherever touched.
- Helps the lymphatics move toxins out of the baby's tissues.
- Aids relaxation.
- Acts as a pain reliever and a sedative by releasing endorphins into the bloodstream.

---

getting started

- Choose an area within your home that is warm, dry and free of draughts.
- Most babies hate being stripped down during the first month, so I recommend laying a towel over the baby's body and exposing only the area you are working on. The weight of the towel will help to soothe the baby and make it easier for you than having to strip down specific body areas at a time.
- Lay the baby on top of one or two folded towels, with the nappy off. Be prepared for accidents – they will happen! – so keep a spare towel, nappy and some wipes nearby.
- The ideal time for massage is after the bath as this minimizes the number of times you are undressing and dressing the baby. Also, the baby's body will be warm and relaxed from the water. Applying oil directly onto the wet skin will help lock in moisture and counteract skin peeling, which is common in the early weeks.
- If possible, some soft background music will help the baby relax.
- Test your baby for allergy to any of the oils used by rubbing a small area onto a patch of skin, such as the upper arm. Any allergic reaction – such as blotching or hives – will usually develop within an hour.
- Apply a good-quality base oil. I always use extra virgin olive oil or sweet almond oil. Exceptionally mild grapeseed oil or organic sunflower oil are recommended for premature babies. (Avoid almond oil if there is a history of epilepsy in the family.)
- Avoid aromatherapy oils until after twelve weeks.
- Take off your watch, rings and any bracelets you are wearing – they could scratch the baby.
- Ensure your hands are warm – run them under warm water first if necessary – and well oiled. Your hands should be able to glide effortlessly. Give them a good shake to relax them before you start.
- Work symmetrically.

- If your baby has a cold, the sniffles or a fever, skip baby massage for a few days.
- If your baby shows any signs of discomfort, stop immediately and scoop him into a cuddle.
- If he just seems disinterested, persevere for up to a few minutes more, concentrating on just one area, such as the foot. Check for any factors that might be contributing to his reluctance – such as a draught, teething, tummy pain, hunger or tiredness. Most babies need four or so sessions before they begin to really enjoy and anticipate the massage, so persevere if you can.
- In the beginning, your massage may only last for five minutes, but it will be easy for you to build on that and work towards 15–20 minute massages.
- Maintain eye contact throughout the massage and sing or talk to him in a soft, low voice.
- Massage can be highly stimulating for your baby, but if you perform gentle, slow moves it can also act as a relaxant, helping him to sleep deeply as a result. He may also want to feed soon after.
- Encourage your partner to perform baby massage as often as possible.

massage routine

Before you lay your hands on the baby, hold up the palms of your hands and show them to him. He will come to recognize this gesture as the beginning of the massage routine.

With the baby lying on his back, perform long, light, sweeping strokes from his head down to his feet. You're simply making him consciously aware of his body. Repeat fifteen times.

FACE

Place both your thumbs on his 'third eye' – the space between his eyebrows – and gently stroke outwards along the upper eyebrow line (Fig. 1). Repeat five times. With your thumbs, and the lightest of touches, trace small circles on his temples (Fig. 2). After five circles, rotate the circles down to the cheekbones and out to the ears. Take the ears between your bent fingers and thumbs and gently squeeze down to the earlobes. Very gently, pull the earlobes down a couple of times.

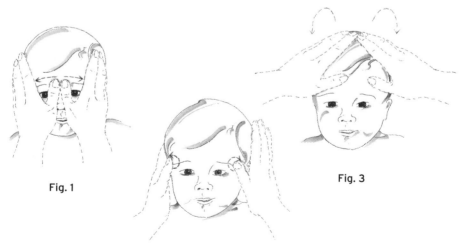

Fig. 1

Fig. 2

Fig. 3

HEAD

The head can be massaged ever so gently with tiny circular movements. First, move around the periphery of the scalp for one or two minutes. Then draw your hands almost off the scalp from the hairline above the forehead at the front of the scalp over and above the top of the head down to the nape of the neck, just three to four times (Fig. 3).

SHOULDERS AND TORSO

Stroke his face and then place your hands on his shoulders and press down very gently so that the shoulders relax beneath the partial weight of your hands. Place your right hand on the baby's right shoulder (Fig. 4) and sweep it down to his left hip bone. Repeat on the other side, then continue the pattern so that the hands criss-cross rhythmically over the torso. This will help the baby feel centred and to join up all the different areas of his body. Repeat ten times. Finish with both hands on the lower tummy.

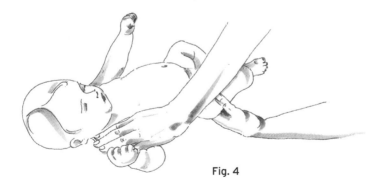

Fig. 4

Keeping both your hands on the centre of his tummy, with your fingers facing up towards his head, sweep up the centre of the torso (Fig. 5). Fan out your fingers as you get to the shoulders so that your hands dip down over the shoulders towards the back. Gently squeeze the large trapezius muscle before gliding your hands back over the shoulders and

Fig. 5

Fig. 6

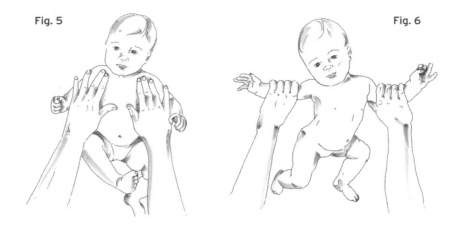

all the way down the arms (Fig. 6). Gently squeeze the palm of the baby's hand and then return your hands to his torso and repeat ten times. Finish with your hands on the centre of his tummy.

TUMMY

With your middle three fingers, rhythmically 'walk' from the lowest part of the abdomen up towards the ribcage (Fig. 7). This gets the baby used to the tummy – a very vulnerable area – being touched. You may find that your baby tenses the tummy initially but this is a natural guarding response. With practice, the baby begins to trust your touch, and after the first few sessions the baby relaxes into your tummy massage. Repeat for one minute. On the whole the tummy massage could last for one to two minutes.

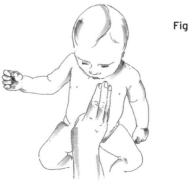

Fig. 7

gentle first year

creative healing tummy massage

Contrary to other massage routines, this creative healing massage avoids going round and round the tummy. Moving the contents of the gut along is actually dealt with in a simple manner by performing light abdominal toning in parallel lines from side to side, moving vertically upwards from the groin, straight up the abdomen, with just a few moves along the direction of flow of the intestinal contents within the ascending, transverse and descending colon. The creative healing constipation spots can be stimulated at every baby massage routine, as explained below.

constipation spots

If your baby is constipated or windy, what really moves the gut along is the stimulation of a special nerve centre that has been described in creative healing as the 'constipation spot'. This nerve centre is located at the two dimples at the top of your baby's buttocks. To perform a constipation treatment you need to place the very end of the tips of your thumbs on each dimple, and then massage upwards with little flicks in an arc shape only half a centimetre in length. Your light flicking strokes should not leave any red marks on the baby's skin.

Massage one arm at a time, gently grasping the whole arm with your cupped hand. Use a generous quantity of oil so that your hand glides smoothly down the entire length of the arm from the level of the armpit all the way down to the hands (Fig. 8).

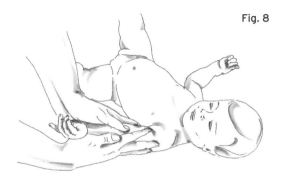

Fig. 8

Alternate your strokes between your baby's right and left arms so that he can sense a rhythm in your massage. Then take each tiny hand and slowly define each finger by stroking each one and stretching it out gently. Then hold each palm with the fingertips of both your hands and gently fan out your fingers and relax your baby's palm. A sort of hand reflexology massage!

LEGS AND FEET

Use both your hands and curl them around the top of your baby's hip, one side at a time. Gently slide your hands down the front and the back of your baby's thigh and leg (Fig. 9), taking care to slide the fingers lightly around the knee. Finish with a gentle squeeze of the foot and repeat ten times. Then move over to the other thigh and leg. The baby's instinct will be to curl the leg in, so gently uncurl the leg and keep it long and soft. If the baby resists uncurling at all, just run your hands over the bent leg for the first few sessions.

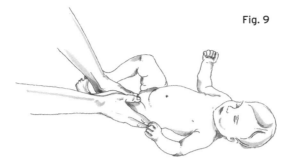

Fig. 9

Let your baby's foot rest in the cup of your hand. With the finger of the same hand, gently massage small circles around the ankle bone for about a minute. Repeat this for about 30 seconds. In reflexology terms this is the area of pelvic lymphatics. So you are getting your baby off to a good start by establishing efficient lymphatic drainage channels.

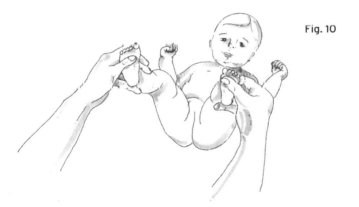

Fig. 10

Then with the pad of your thumb, gently press long lines up the soles of the baby's foot, finishing at the toes (Fig. 10). Repeat for 20 seconds.

Very, very gently, take each tiny toe and pass it through your fingers. The movements are minute.

Repeat this foot sequence on the other leg.

If at all possible, pass your baby through some incense that you can burn in a clay pot. Nowadays you can buy charcoal discs from most new-age stores. These light up easily and glow like embers. You can then sprinkle a few grains of the frankincense resin on top. This will generate a cloud of sweet-smelling incense – just like in church services. Almost all homes in southern India generate clouds of incense both morning and night. The incense-carrying holder is passed through all the rooms of the house concentrating on the corners, supposedly driving out negative energy.

play

what is baby play?

If you were to ask adults how babies play, they would probably say something like chewing their toes, pushing a ball or rolling around like happy hippos. And they'd be right. Except, that behaviour is performed by six-month-old babies! For the first twelve weeks, your tiny newborn has more in common with the unborn foetus.

In the first three months, your baby cannot sit up or hold his head up. He cannot as yet grab a toy, point to it, or once he's got it, let it go. This has far-reaching implications on how you play with your newborn, and it's a big, big shock for the first-time parent, who expected to go straight into peek-a-boo.

how do i play with my newborn?

So what exactly are you expected to do? Well, the biggest thing for you is redefining your idea of what constitutes play. When we think of the games we played as children, we remember the results: laughter and fun, elements of surprise, and thrills of the chase. We don't see the developmental milestones around which these games have been built up. For example, we think banging a saucepan with a wooden spoon is at worst noise and at best a precursor to musicality, rather than an early conception of cause and effect (if I bang this pan, it'll make a noise). Equally, we remember hide and seek for the thrill of being hunted, rather than introducing us to the concept of object permanence (something still existing even though we can't see it.). Singing 'Round and Round the Garden' may be a pretty story with a big tickle, but it also teaches us about anticipation.

play stages

The journey of play in the first three months basically travels from you (yes, you are the entertainment) to their bodies and finally to toys. And there's really only one rule to follow: repeat, repeat, ad infinitum. If you think you're boring your baby doing the same thing over and over, think again. Each time you repeat an action he learns a little more about it; and when he has finally mastered it, that's when he'll turn away in boredom.

THE FIRST MONTH: BONDING PLAY

In the first month, your baby is absorbing all the alien sounds, smells and sights surrounding him. He can only see as far as 12 inches – the distance between mother and baby's faces when the baby is on the breast. His biggest focus is learning who to trust and rely on – bonding – so play in this first month should centre on facilitating that. Any activity that allows him to study you – your voice, your face, your smell, your touch – is ideal:

In the first month, your baby is absorbing all the alien sounds, smells and sights surrounding him.

- Let him learn your voice through songs and rhymes.
- You can read books to him and he'll be fascinated by the inflections and cadence of your voice.
- Sway him in your arms as you sing and dance to your favourite songs.
- Cuddle him cheek to cheek.
- Prop up a clear photo of yourself in his cot for him to examine.
- Make funny faces for him to study (his brain will be storing absolutely every single one for hard-wiring later on).

- And touch him lovingly – through massage, tickles or just relaxing strokes – whilst you look into his eyes.

THE SECOND MONTH: DOING PLAY

By the second month, his anxiety levels will have dropped and he'll be more placid during his waking moments. Play during this month gradually becomes less about you and more about what his body allows him to do: His eyesight will have improved although his focus is still soft. For this reason, bold single images in colourful board books really come into their own and will hold your baby's gaze for longer and longer. Regular periods spent lying on his tummy (even if only for a few minutes at a time at first) provide good bursts of physical exercise and will sometimes – surprisingly, for both you and him – lead to rolling, which is always greeted with much excitement. And because he now knows your voice, he will begin to remember and recognize familiar tunes, so make sure you have one or two 'special' songs that you sing every day, without fail. They can be sung at set times, such as just before naps, or at random. Most babies have a good sense of humour, and clownish behaviour of silly faces is usually to their taste. Repeating words that begin with 'S' will also encourage your baby to smile, because your baby is, at heart, a mimic and enunciating the letter S brings the mouth into a natural, faint smile. You'll probably giggle too at the ridiculous combinations you dream up – 'My silly sparrow swallowed a slinky snowflake', and so on.

The most exciting development in the second month has to be the advent of gummy smiles.

By the third month, your baby will be much more robust and really enjoying exploring his physicality, and you will probably find yourself in more natural and recognizable play categories. Tickling, clapping and blowing are all met with delight, as is being held above you and then gently brought down to your face for a kiss. During playtime, give samplers of different sensations which will delight the skin and nerve endings – tickle him with a furry ball or flutter your eyelashes on his cheeks for butterfly kisses. Best of all, shower him with kisses.

Once the baby is twelve weeks old, you will finally be able to introduce some toys to initiate the grabbing technique that will be developing. Once that is in action, rattles, soft toys and baby gyms will take some pressure off you, as what were previously your props now thoroughly absorb him in their own right.

In all, the art of playing with a newborn baby can be creative and intimate. And it's also crucial – it's through play that your baby learns, refines and thrives. It's excellent fun. So enjoy!

The art of playing with a newborn baby can be creative and intimate. It's also crucial – and excellent fun.

baby care

weeks one to three

- If possible, make an appointment to see a cranio-sacral therapist in the next three weeks. Lying for long hours on a flat surface can create a flat head that a cranial therapist can correct as the baby develops. Also, the suckling impulse can create a tightness at the cranial base that could lead to colic and perhaps sleep disorders. A cranial therapist is trained to look for these stresses and strains and correct them. Regular sessions of cranio-sacral therapy can be a big comfort to the baby and ensure that all the developmental milestones are met magnificently.
- Feed on demand for the first two weeks to really establish your milk supply. After the first fortnight you might find that the baby begins to feed naturally at two- to four-hourly intervals. Let the baby sleep as long as he wants at night and wait until he wakes for feeds.
- The umbilical stump may be off by now, but if it is still holding on, it might be black and shrivelled. If it is red, or looks as if it has pus on it, see your health visitor to check for infection. Keep it clean with twice-daily wipes with antiseptic cotton wool and a solution of 20ml water with one drop of tea tree oil.
- If your baby is colicky, 'cycling' his legs can help move trapped wind in the lower gut. You may well find he enjoys it so much that this could become an early way of playing together. (See page 19 for Ayurvedic baby stretches.)
- Be sure to support your baby's head every time you lift him.
- Swaddle the baby for sleeps in the first month. Once he starts to wriggle free, half-swaddle him (see page 10) for a couple of weeks. When he is happily going to sleep with arms outstretched (from five weeks onwards), put him in a baby sleeping bag or, better still, a baby hammock if you can get hold of one.
- Place your baby to sleep on a baby sheepskin in the winter months, or a soft cotton blanket.

- Gradually introduce baths. You could add a couple of drops of Rescue Remedy to the bath water to create a calming effect.
- During bathing, do a few minutes of baby floating. This will relax the baby's body and encourage him to maintain eye contact for longer than usual, promoting good bonding. Put a few drops of Rescue Remedy into the bath water at about 34 degrees centigrade (most babies prefer a slightly warmer bath of 36 degrees centigrade). With one hand on the back of your baby's head and the other beneath his bottom, gently float the baby backwards and forwards in the water. Ideally, sing a lullaby as you do this. Try to keep the baby's ears out of the water and the umbilical stump dry (although if it does get wet simply pat dry with a separate, clean towel afterwards). If the baby makes a fuss, you can get in and gently cradle him in the water next to you, keeping his arms and legs close and tucked up. After a couple of sessions, he'll begin to feel happier with his limbs outstretched. Some babies may cry for the first couple of times as they hate having their clothes off, but they soon enjoy the feeling of weightlessness.
- Warm your baby's towel and sleep suit on the radiator – an instant soother upon coming out of the water.
- It is a good idea to consult a homeopath in the first few weeks after birth as they will advise you about how to protect your baby and discuss immunization issues.
- In the first month, playtime really is face time and skin touching. Hold your baby close and let him examine your face. He will be entranced by your eyes blinking, your eyebrows raised, your nose wrinkling, your smile and shiny teeth. Poke out your tongue as he may well copy you. Make your eyes wide. Let him see how expressive faces can be. Remember, you'll also look very different to your baby if you wear your hair back in a ponytail or put on a shower cap, so make sure he gets to examine you each time you make an adjustment to your appearance.
- Keep up with your 'special' song that you sing to him every day,

which is just for the two of you. Encourage the baby's father to sing his own special song every day too.

- As well as taking the baby for walks in the pram, occasionally carry him in a baby sling with adequate head support. Even though your hands will be free, still cuddle him really close and kiss the top of his head. He'll feel safe, deeply loved and comforted by the familiar sense of your physical motion.

weeks four to seven

- In the second month, your baby's limbs are more outstretched and you can introduce floating on his tummy. Support the chest with one hand, gently supporting the baby's chin and making sure the baby's face is above the level of the water. Hold your other hand beneath the hips. Slowly move your baby backwards and forwards, always watching the face and making sure his mouth and nose are above water.

- You can follow the now well-established daily bath with a daily massage routine too. I advise my mothers to follow the routine detailed earlier in this chapter (see page 90), which is devised specifically for newborns, but vary the pattern each day, and some sessions may be shorter than others. But try to make a priority of doing a light massage for at least five to ten minutes as part of your touch therapy.

- After three weeks, start to place the baby on his tummy, with arms forward and palms flat on the floor, and with a firm pillow over his feet so that he can lever against it and lift his upper body more easily. These sessions may be as short as a minute to begin with but will gradually build up to about five to ten minutes at a time. Make sure the baby is on a level surface (hips lower than the shoulders) and that a folded towel or padded mat is placed beneath the baby's face as he might drop his head sharply to the floor quite often until he's got more strength. Be present all the time during this exercise.

- Between four and six weeks, you'll be rewarded with the first gummy smile —and, like labour, you'll know when it's the real thing. You can read the smile in your baby's eyes, and you'll instinctively smile back before you've even processed this little miracle.
- When you are running your baby's bath, remove all his clothes and let him lie naked, wriggling and luxuriating upon a fleecy blanket or sheepskin. Place an absorbent towel under the bottom as the newfound freedom from his nappy may well prompt him to do a little wee! Total nakedness for about five to ten minutes is very pleasurable for your baby and really stimulates the skin.
- Your baby's head will still need to be supported when being held against your tummy. An alternative holding position is the Tiger in the Tree (see page 77), which particularly calms down colicky babies.
- After six weeks, your baby will be getting strong enough for the Throne position. This is good for babies who like to be held a lot. Place your baby in a sitting position with his back against your tummy. Rest his bottom across your bent arm and drape your other arm across the tummy, securing your baby's position at all times. This position keeps him secure, supports the head and gives him a good view of everything around.
- On the rare occasion when you have to go in to wake your baby, rouse him from sleep by gently stroking and kissing the temples. This is the most vulnerable area of the head, so deliberately directing love and gentleness there will instinctively make your baby feel safe and secure with you, promoting bonding.
- In the second month, nappy changes become an opportunity for playtime too. Gently shake and stretch the legs; squeeze and kiss the thighs (which should really be chunking up by now); blow soft raspberries onto his tummy as you sing your special song.
- Increase the amount of 'face time' you share with your baby by lying on the sofa with your knees bent and your back propped up. Lay the baby in the crook of your lap and sing songs, hold his hands, tickle his little feet and stroke his hair, face and cheeks.

- Your baby is still learning to sense the difference between your body and theirs. So during playtime give samplers of different sensations which will delight the skin and nerve endings – tickle with a furry ball; flutter your eyelashes on your baby's cheeks and give butterfly kisses.

weeks eight to twelve

- Interactive rhymes like 'Round and Round the Garden', 'This Little Piggy', 'Incy Wincy Spider' and 'Pat-a-cake' show your baby other more remote areas of his body – such as the armpits or toes – and begin to introduce the idea of anticipation.
- One of the big developmental milestones of this age group is learning to grasp or reach. Encourage this by gently shaking a rattle. It can be a wooden bead rattle or a soft toy one, but the noise and sight will intrigue your baby. The synapses in his brain will make a connection that will enable him to stretch out an arm and get to investigate the cause of so much excitement.
- As your baby becomes stronger, help develop head control with the following exercise: lay the baby on his back and take hold of his hands in yours. *Very* slowly pull your baby upwards into a sitting position. Initially, the head will fall back but as the neck muscles get stronger, head holding will get better. Practise daily. Be very careful when you return him to the lying down position and make sure that the neck is straight and in alignment with the back and spine.
- Continue the tummy mat work (see page 103). By now your baby will be able to hold her head for significant periods and look around. Prop a plastic baby mirror in front of your baby's face – babies love to look at themselves.
- White noise is intrinsically soothing, so sit your baby in front of the washing machine – babies are intrigued by the bubbles and whirling motion, especially on the spin cycle!

two to twelve weeks

- A bouncy chair with suspended toy arch is also fun (and helpful too if you have other children to entertain). Change the toys regularly to keep up different stimulations and hang them at 'batting' distance so that he can practise reaching.
- If you have long hair, lean over and let it hang forward over your face. Your baby will love being so close to your face and being enclosed in your scent.
- Encourage your baby to copy you – try waving or clapping.

vaccination

Vaccination is a controversial topic. For every trial which reports no adverse effects, there is a counter claim testifying to their harm. The decision is personal, involved and emotional and I do not think, within the scope of this book, that I can give a definitive direction on this topic. But what I can do is show you what complementary options are available to you, should you want them.

Parents often ask if there is a homeopathic alternative to conventional vaccinations. Here is some advice from Lynne Howard, the Homeopath who practises with me at my clinic:

vaccination - notes from a homeopath

Whether or not to vaccinate your child can be a difficult decision for some parents. It may be helpful to consult a homeopath who offers vaccination counselling, as she will be able to discuss the alternative ways in which homeopathic treatment can be used to support your decision.

Some homeopaths offer remedies relating to a list of specific diseases in a scheduled programme, in the belief that these may help prevent these diseases. As yet there is little evidence that this is helpful.

The best course of action is to keep your child as healthy as possible whether you give them vaccinations or not. Homeopaths can treat your child with constitutional remedies which experience tells us can raise their level of health, help treat any tendencies to chronic diseases such as allergies and make them less susceptible to becoming ill with recurrent acute infections such as ear infections or repeated coughs. Acute infections such as fever and sore throats are often the body's attempt to stimulate its own healing powers, and help it heal itself of the tendency to develop more chronic diseases such as asthma. Your homeopath can advise you on how best to treat the numerous acute infections that your child experiences, in order that symptoms are not simply suppressed back into the body.

If you decide to vaccinate your child, your homeopath may give a remedy that is made from the vaccine. This has been found through clinical experience to help symptoms that may have arisen after having the vaccination.

Whether or not your child is vaccinated, during an epidemic of a childhood illness your homeopath can give you a remedy that may help prevent your child having the disease. Your homeopath may give you several of these epidemic remedies to keep at home in case of need.

In the event that your child becomes ill with a childhood disease there are many homeopathic remedies that may help your child recover from the illness more quickly and with less discomfort.

mother

getting your body back

I always tell my mothers that the physicality of having a baby is not spread over nine months, but twelve. For three months after the birth your body is recovering from the effects of pregnancy.

the first six weeks

In the first six weeks after birth, your body is healing from labour and childbirth. During this phase:

- Your lochia (postnatal bleeding) slowly gets lighter and then stops.
- Your uterus, cervix and fallopian tubes involute back to their pre-pregnant shape and size.
- If you have had an episiotomy or a Caesarean section, your scars heal completely and internal bruising fades.
- Breastfeeding becomes established and the initial engorgement disappears.

BIRTH RECOVERY TREATMENTS

In the first week, I advise a creative healing 'female treatment' to provide immediate support to those areas of the body placed under intense strain during the birth process. The heart and uterus are both involuting rapidly, and after the birth of the baby there will be rapid changes in the circulating blood volume. Three to four litres of excess fluid will be urinated out of the body within the first 24 hours, and this alone contributes to a feeling of lightness after the birth. The creative healing treatments in week one help with this flushing out process, prevent congestion in the tissues and help to minimize shock. (See Chapter 1 for further information on female treatments.)

The treatments in weeks two to six have less urgency and are more concerned with assisting the body's natural healing process. This means using Bowen and cranio-sacral therapy to reset muscles and neuro-muscular pathways that might have got overstretched or misaligned during birthing. Creative healing is amazing for easing tension out of sore, tired muscles – such as shoulders, lower back and thighs – which were involved in the pushing stage. Reflexology is known to speed excretion and has a stimulating effect on the kidneys and the gut. It is also relaxing and promotes deep sleep, which is especially useful when the mother has to catch a deep sleep between feeds. Warm oil massages soothe the central nervous system after the agitation of the birth and balance the hormonal flux to support lactation for breastfeeding.

weeks seven to twelve

Working alongside this and beyond, into the second six weeks, your body is still recovering and overcoming some of the physiological effects of pregnancy. This is known as 'puerperium' and is the postnatal phase when all the organs that hypertrophied (enlarged) in pregnancy, such as the womb, heart and kidneys, return to their original state. (My postnatal toning-up CD talks you through a deep relaxation and aspects of postnatal physical recovery, see Resources.)

Naturally, this physical restoration is not happening alone. You are on a steep learning curve of acquiring new mothering skills, as well as adjusting to the huge emotional shift of becoming a mother and the restrictions this places on your time, movements and sense of self. If your world has changed irrevocably, your body hasn't (though that may be hard to believe at the moment!). It's just that it'll be a while longer before your body returns to its original size.

In the second half of this post-partum period, we are concerned with treating the longer-standing effects of the pregnancy. For example, I recommend Bowen at eight weeks, as the baby may have presented asymmetrically in the pelvis, but rather flipped to one side or the other during the later stage of pregnancy, causing uneven pressure within the mother's pelvis and abdomen. This means that one side of the body will have been working harder than the other for a sizeable portion of the pregnancy. As a result, there will be some muscular imbalances that need to be rectified, and some neurological pathways to be reset.

A creative healing 'digestive tune-up' counteracts the slowing effect of the pregnancy hormone progesterone on the digestive tract. This and other creative healing treatments can prevent heartburn, indigestion and constipation, whilst a back treatment will help to tone up and tighten the ligaments of the back and reverse progesterone's birth-orientated loosening effect on the sacral and pelvic muscles.

My favourite postnatal treatments are Ayurvedic massages. These can, in the long run, nourish and rebuild the mother's tissues. The oils are medicinal and specially formulated to tone up the mother's internal organs, as well as the muscular-skeletal system. Traditionally, these massages are given to the mother at home every day for forty days in the post-partum period.

Another option is to listen to my postnatal toning-up CD daily. This talks you through returning your body to its pre-pregnant levels, and galvanizes you into becoming even more toned than before (see Resources).

cosmetic tip: waist-trimming panty

You may well find you've changed bra size after your baby is born and you have stopped breastfeeding. This is because as the baby grows up into the abdominal cavity, your ribcage is gently expanded and forced out to create room for the baby. This subtle process occurs very gradually – some mothers find they ache in their ribs during the latter part of the pregnancy – and the ribs do not naturally 'fall' back into place afterwards but have to be 'trained' back in. I prescribe a special support panty which applies gentle pressure on the lower ribs and coaxes them back to their original position. It is soft and very discreet as it can be worn under normal clothes during the day. The French have long sworn by this custom, and now so does Hollywood (see Resources).

ayurvedic diagnosis

Those mothers who followed the gentle birth method will already be familiar with the Ayurvedic model I use to diagnose potential problems and weak spots in each mother's pregnancy.

For those of you new to the gentle method, Ayurveda is the ancient, and highly-respected, holistic doctrine which is commonly used for treating disease and illness in India, where I grew up and trained as a doctor. Even now, it is consulted by many people alongside mainstream Western medical practice, and is gaining popularity around the world.

Ayurveda, literally translated, means 'life science'. It purports that the root of disease lies in the body's natural equilibrium being out of balance.

In Western physiology, your body type can be classified into one of three main groupings – endormorph, ectomorph and mesomorph – which signify certain body types and characteristics. In Ayurveda, your constitution (known as *prakruti*) is determined by three similar classifications, known as *doshas*. These are *vata*, *pitta* and *kapha*. Each *prakruti* is defined by specific physical traits and behaviourisms which may make it more prone to certain imbalances – and therefore illnesses – than others.

I use this diagnostic model with great success with the mothers who come to my London clinic. Just as it is useful for predicting – and therefore avoiding – certain complications in pregnancy, the same can be done for the post-partum period.

which body type are you?

Below is a chart that will help determine your *prakruti*, and this will help you to tailor your physical recovery more specifically. However, it takes many years to become practised in Ayurvedic teaching, and it is not the intention of the chart here to be comprehensive or rigid. Most people are a combination of two *doshas* rather than just one, so work from your dominant *dosha* and merely look over your secondary one to bear certain aspects in mind. If you would like a more detailed and prescribed diagnosis, I strongly recommend consulting a respected Ayurvedic practitioner (see Resources).

Please use the chart on pages 113–16 to find your predominant *dosha* at the moment (the immediate postnatal phase). Your answers may be quite different from those you would give at other times in your life.

Read each of the following statements and score them individually on a scale of one to five, according to how accurate they are for you (0 = completely inappropriate, 5 = an accurate description). Add up the scores for each section – *vata*, *pitta* and *kapha* – and analyse the final scores to find your predominant *dosha*.

	0	1	2	3	4	5

VATA

I am slim and don't gain weight easily	
My appetite is irregular	
I have an erratic lifestyle	
I am a dreamer and don't usually finish projects	
I have irregular bowel movements and am prone to constipation	
I get cold hands and feet	
I am talkative	
I get anxious and worried easily	
I am creative and like to express myself creatively	
I prefer warm weather	
My skin is cool, rough and dry	
I am not very strong and lose stamina easily	
I walk quickly	
I am a light sleeper	

	0	1	2	3	4	5

I learn easily but I also forget easily	
I get a lot of wind	
I am moody	
I find it difficult to make decisions	
I have short bursts of energy	
My menstrual cycles are irregular and I have period pains with associated headaches	
TOTAL SCORE	

PITTA

My dreams are in colour	
I eliminate my food quickly through my gut	
I have a good memory	
I grasp things very well	
I prefer cooler climates	
I can be bossy and forceful	
I become irritable if I skip a meal	
I eat quite a lot	
I sleep soundly	
I have regular bowel movements	

	0	1	2	3	4	5

I have good stamina for physical activities	
I am a perfectionist	
I don't like hot environments	
I sweat a lot	
People consider me very stubborn and I get angry very easily	
I criticize others and myself easily	
I have a very busy life	
I have a medium build	
My eyes are sharp and bright	
I like ice creams and cold drinks	
TOTAL SCORE	

KAPHA

I am of big build	
I am muscular	
I prefer warm weather	
My hair is thick and lustrous	
My appetite is good and I enjoy food	
I learn slowly, but I have a good long-term memory	

	0	1	2	3	4	5

I have slow digestion; this makes me feel heavy after a meal	
I walk with slow, measured steps	
I like a relaxed life	
I have regular bowel movements	
When I menstruate I have regular, normal periods	
I gain weight easily – people call me plump	
I have a pleasant voice	
I am calm by nature	
I love sleeping and sleep deeply	
My skin is cool and oily	
I don't like cold weather	
I am good-natured and nothing seems to bother me	
I am possessive	
I wake up slowly and I don't like waking up	
TOTAL SCORE	

ayurvedic treatments

Typical Characteristics

- Lean, small frame
- Dry skin
- Mentally excitable
- Weak constitution – prone to colds and illnesses
- Poor circulation
- Poor digestion with tendency to constipation
- Low energy
- May experience fainting
- *Vata* in balance: alert and spontaneous
- *Vata* out of balance: worried and experiences mood swings

How to Balance Vata

Exercise

- Exercise in moderation, as the *vata* mother is rather weak. Engage in mild to moderate exercise only. Walking and swimming are good.

Food

- Eat three to four regular light meals a day, preferably containing a representation of all the tastes: salty, sour, bitter, sweet, pungent and astringent.
- Avoid snacks between meals.
- Choose clear soups or chicken or fish soups.
- Avoid cheese as *vata* mothers have poor digestion.

Herbs

The following herbs can balance *vata*:

- Black pepper
- Dill seeds
- Cumin seeds
- Basil leaves
- Parsley
- Ginger

Physical Treatments

- Massage with oils can be amazingly effective in reducing excessive *vata*.
- Self-massage or being massaged by your partner on a regular basis, for twenty to forty minutes, is recommended. Suitable oils are virgin olive oil, sesame oil or a sesame-based Ayurvedic compound oil such as dhanwanthari oil.
- Essential oils can also be used to reduce *vata* – try lavender, rose or jasmine oil. Use four to ten drops in 20ml base oil. This can be used for self-massage or by a practitioner during general or creative healing massage.
- Reflexology reduces *vata*, calms the mind and gives mental clarity. It also improves digestion and speeds up gut motility, thereby relieving constipation.

PITTA MOTHERS

Typical Characteristics

- Skin redness
- Medium-size body frame
- Slightly oily skin
- Fluid retention
- Angry
- Mentally irritable and edgy
- Quick tempered

- Intolerant of others' behaviour
- Experiences skin burning sensations
- Feels too hot all the time
- Can't tolerate hot weather
- Hates closed environments
- Prone to feeling faint
- Prone to increased sweating
- Good memory
- Sound sleeper
- *Pitta* in balance: perceptive and intense
- *Pitta* out of balance: angry, impatient and frustrated

How to Balance Pitta

Food
- Avoid hot and spicy foods like pepper, chillies and garlic. Acidic and sour foods aggravate *pitta* so avoid vinegar, salad creams, pickles and sour things in general.
- No alcohol.
- Most vegetables are good – cucumber, marrows and pumpkins are ideal; beetroots and carrots are very cooling and recommended.
- Eat grains such as rice, millet, corn and oats in moderation (once a week).
- Cut out tomatoes. If you must eat them, restrict it to only once a week. Tomato is very acidic. Cooked tomato is worse than raw tomato.
- Coconut is very good for reducing *pitta*.
- Apples are very good but avoid citrus fruits.
- Having a banana once a week can reduce *pitta*.
- Vegetable soups with herbs are very soothing.
- Milk is cooling and good for reducing *pitta*. Ideally it should be goat's milk.

Herbs
- Choose cooling herbs like coriander in food.

Treatments

- Creative healing massage includes a cooling procedure that is good for counteracting excessive *pitta*.
- For massage, use essential oils like lavender, jasmine and sandalwood. The recommended base oils for *pitta* are sesame oil and coconut oil.
- Have a milk bath (cow's or goat's milk) as Cleopatra did. Simply add some milk to your bath water.
- Take a flower bath, with petals floating in the bath – try rose or jasmine flower.
- It should also be noted that *pitta* mothers are more prone to postnatal depression. This can be prevented by keeping to the *pitta* protocol for diet and treatments.

KAPHA MOTHERS

Typical Characteristics

- Large frame
- Oily skin
- Gains weight easily
- A tendency for water retention
- Drawn to sweet foods
- Digestive sluggishness
- Passive
- Calm, steady
- Lethargic
- Slow to be irritated
- Heavy sleeper
- *Kapha* in balance: strong and calm
- *Kapha* out of balance: dull and lethargic

How to Balance Kapha

Exercise
- All forms of exercise benefit the *kapha* mother.

Food
- Do not eat anything white or high in carbohydrate – avoid toast, bread, potatoes and rice pudding.
- Avoid pasta, cakes, crisps and ice creams.
- Avoid beef, pork and lamb. Chicken is allowed – two small portions per week.
- Choose spicy foods.
- Eat lots of green vegetables and light clear soups.

Treatments
- Warm baths are very beneficial – add a few drops of basil essential oil as this activates your endorphins and improves your mood.
- Other essential oils that can reduce *kapha* and lift your mood are eucalyptus, camphor, neroli, tea tree, juniper and fennel. Use in massage oils, or add to your bath.
- Have regular lymphatic drainage massage (creative healing massage is very efficient for lymphatic drainage).
- Reflexology is great for reducing *kapha*. Focus on the lymphatic drainage reflex areas on the feet to make sure the lymph drainage channels are kept clear.

how to reduce postnatal kapha and vata

Most mothers have increased *kapha* and *vata* in the immediate postnatal period. The following recommendations for pacifying *vata* and *kapha* may, therefore, be helpful. I have listed them in order of importance.

1 **Avoid cold drinks and foods in the immediate postnatal phase and for the first two weeks.** I worry about some of my mothers who, having followed my 'no wheat and no sugar' policy during pregnancy, make a beeline for ice cream as soon as they have given birth! Eating this will chill the stomach and pancreas and have a negative effect on digestion. This will lead to bloating caused by food stagnating and fermenting within the gut. It is important to consume water only at room temperature or warmer. I hope that midwives nationwide will become informed that iced water is not good for mothers during labour or in the immediate postnatal phase.

2 **Drink rasam, a special spicy 'pepper water' from India and Sri Lanka, to warm the digestive system.** It is beneficial to drink rasam in the immediate postnatal phase, and even within twenty-four hours of birth. Light and watery with minimal fat, rasam is full of spices to get the digestive juices flowing. All the ingredients have a warming and toning effect on the stomach and the entire digestive tract. This remedies the distended bowel that most of my mothers exhibit throughout their pregnancies. (In creative healing, intestinal distension is treated with a full digestive tune-up at least once a month during the pregnancy and in the postnatal months.)

Recipe for Rasam

All these ingredients are easily available in local supermarkets.

1 clove of garlic, chopped or crushed
½ an onion, finely chopped
1 teaspoon of sesame or sunflower oil
½ teaspoon each of cumin, coriander and fennel seeds
4 peppercorns
3 cloves
5cm (2-inch) stick of cinnamon
1 whole dried red chilli
2 pinches of asafoetida*
6 dried or fresh curry leaves
¼ teaspoon of tamarind paste dissolved in a pint of water

* Asafoetida is an astringent flavouring agent. Actually a resin in powdered form, it is popular in Iran, Afghanistan and India.

1 Roast the garlic and the chopped onion in a teaspoon of sesame or sunflower oil.
2 Add all the ingredients except for the tamarind water. Fry for about two minutes till a lovely aroma arises.
3 Pour in the pint of tamarind water. Allow the whole mixture to come to the boil and let it simmer for about six minutes.

3 **Take a special herbal tonic called Dashamoolarishtam.** This pacifies all three *doshas* and is a great uterine tonic as well. Available to buy from most Ayurvedic pharmacies.
4 **Take Jeerarishtam to encourage breast milk production.** The main ingredient is fennel seeds. You can make an infusion at home (see page 38).

5 **Eat jackfruit curry.** This is traditionally given to postnatal mothers in southern India and Sri Lanka to enhance breast milk production. The jackfruit grows to massive proportions, comically attached to the trunk of the large jackfruit tree. The local people cut the unripe fruit into small pieces and make a curry that they say has much more nutritional value than a beef curry. Jackfruit can be bought in Asian supermarkets.

6 **Take the herb Ashwagandha (*Withania somnifera*), an excellent stress reliever.** This can be taken by the mother two weeks after giving birth, for about six weeks, if she needs an energy boost. An amazing remedy for tired mothers and fathers, it boosts the immune system and metabolism, and increases libido and physical energy. It is also known to reduce inflammation in cases of arthritis and myositis. Happily, this herb is available from Solgar, and can be found in health-food stores in the UK. The dosage is one capsule twice a day.

7 **Drink baladi choornam.** I recommend this drink to mothers during their pregnancy. It is also a *vata* pacifier and as such is very useful in the postnatal phase up to three months. (Can be taken while breastfeeding.)

8 **Take dhanwantharam pills (baby pills).** These are suitable all the way through pregnancy and postnatally (including during breastfeeding). They are generally very strengthening and good for digestion, and are available from www.gentlebirthmethod.com.

ayurvedic baby diagnosis

Yes, even babies can be predominantly *vata*, *pitta* or *kapha*. Find out your baby's body type by reading the chart on page 125 and circling the tendencies your baby exhibits.

If you circle more than four in any one section, your baby is likely to belong to that body type. (It is rare to exhibit the characteristics of just one *dosha*. Most babies have a mixed *dosha*, similar to most adults.)

	Vata babies	Kapha babies	Pitta babies
Bones	Long and thin	Short	Optimum length
Body Weight	Underweight	Overweight	Optimum weight
Skin texture	Dry and flaky	Moist	Skin eruptions
Hair	Thin and dry	Lots of hair - looks oily	Average hair
Sleep patterns	Erratic	Sleeps deeply	Balanced sleep
Feeding pattern	Hurried and not satisfied	Long and sustained	Moderate
Stools	Tendency to constipation	Normal consistency	Loose and watery
TOTAL SCORE			

SIMPLE AYURVEDIC REMEDIES

Vata Babies

- **Baby massage**. To balance *vata*, the best treatment is baby massage with cured sesame oil. This is a lighter version of the sesame oil that is commonly available in southern India and Sri Lanka. The oil is warmed to body temperature, and the direction of Ayurvedic baby massage resembles the creative healing baby massage pattern I advocate. The limbs are massaged in a downward direction at both the front and the back of the body. The upper half of the baby's trunk is massaged with arc-shaped movements on either side of the trunk, starting above the level of the waist and spreading out towards the shoulders.

- **Floral baths.** Give the baby a bath (at about 34 degrees centigrade) in which you suspend fresh or dried jasmine flowers, if available. What luxury!

REMEDIES FOR THE VATA BABY'S MOTHER

- **Massage.** Massage yourself with cured sesame or mustard seed oil.
- **Drink coriander tea.** (See following recipe.) This seems to be the panacea for all the different *dosha* mothers postnatally!

Recipe for Coriander Tea

- Roast a tablespoon of dry coriander seeds in a dry saucepan over a moderate heat till they emit a lovely aroma.
- Add two cups of water and a tablespoon of fresh or dried ginger and simmer for ten to twenty minutes.
- Strain and drink. You can sweeten it with maple syrup.

The Pitta Baby

- **Floral baths.** Suspend rose petals in the bath water (at about 34 degrees centigrade). If possible, use home-grown rose petals that have not been sprayed with pesticides. Otherwise source some good-quality rose water or rose hydrolat (a form of rose water available on the internet) and add a few drops to the bath water.

Remedies for the Pitta Baby's Mother

- **Coriander tea.** Again, the mother benefits from drinking coriander tea, as above.
- **Rose or jasmine infusion.** It's also beneficial for the mother to drink an infusion of rose or jasmine petals (organic).
- **Ayurvedic massage.** Use dhanwantharam oil on its own, or mixed with equal quantities of mustard oil or coconut oil. If an Ayurvedic practitioner or specific oils are not available, you can perform self-massage on a daily basis with equal quantities of coconut oil mixed with mustard oil or cured sesame oil. Warm the oil for maximum benefit.

The Kapha Baby

- **Warm oil baby massage.** This will move the lymph and increase the metabolic rate. *Kapha* babies are prone to chest infections so it is good to keep them in warm environments and give them lots of body contact.

Remedies for the Kapha baby's mother

- **Coriander tea.** Again, she needs to drink coriander tea made as above but with twice as much ginger. Ideally, she should drink this at least twice a day as it reduces mucus within the body.
- **Warm oil massage.** She will also benefit from massage given in a comfortably warm environment as it is aimed at lymphatic drainage. She must dress warmly, even in the summer, as she is also prone to chest infections.

ayurvedic recipes

The following recipes are for dishes that are easy to digest and nourishing in the postnatal phase.

Recipe for Ginger Infusion with Medicinal Herbs

This traditional remedy for postnatal mothers has warming properties. Even in the tropics, mothers are advised to keep warm and have warming remedies after birth.

1 tablespoon of dried ginger, crushed
3 whole peppercorns
½ a teaspoon of fennel
1 clove of garlic, peeled
1 teaspoon of lovage seeds

Grind all the ingredients together, then add a teaspoon of maple syrup to a teaspoon of this mixture and eat it bit by bit, savouring and swallowing it.

Recipe for Chicken Roast

1 tablespoon of butter
1 tablespoon of sunflower oil
1 teaspoon of fresh ground ginger
3 cloves of fresh garlic, ground
4 peppercorns
¼ teaspoon of ground cinnamon
200g of chicken, preferably organic, cut into bite-sized pieces
Salt and pepper

1 Put the butter and oil in a pan.
2 When the butter has melted, put in the ground ginger, garlic, peppercorns and cinnamon.
3 Add the chicken pieces.
4 Cook, covered, over a low heat till the meat is cooked. Stir occasionally.
5 Season with salt and pepper and cook till all the liquid evaporates and you get dry-fried chicken.

Recipe for Chicken/Lamb/Beef Soup

2 large onions, diced
200g of chicken, lamb or beef, cut into small pieces
1 carrot, sliced
Salt to taste
Pepper to taste
3 cloves of garlic, peeled
3 cups of water

Cook all the ingredients together in a pot until the soup reduces to half the quantity. Liquidize and eat.

Recipe for Garlic Curry

This is delicious! Please avoid red chilli powder in this recipe, and stick to ground black pepper.

1 tablespoon of sunflower oil

¼ teaspoon of mustard seeds

1 tablespoon of urud dhal (a kind of lentil with a black skin – available at Indian grocery stores)

2 medium onions, chopped finely

6–8 curry leaves, fresh or dry (if not available substitute with a few sprigs of coriander leaves)

50–60 cloves of garlic, peeled

1 teaspoon cumin (jeera) powder

¼ teaspoon of ground black pepper

Tamarind water (dissolve a tablespoon of tamarind paste in a cup of warm water)

Salt to taste (usually about 1½ teaspoons)

1 Heat the oil. Add the mustard seeds and urud dhal and stir-fry with a wooden spatula. When the seeds begin to pop, add the onions, curry leaves and the garlic and continue to sauté the whole mixture.
2 Next add the cumin and pepper powder and continue to sauté for a few more minutes.
3 Then stir in the tamarind water and let it simmer for a few minutes.
4 Finally, add the salt and cook till the garlic is soft.

menu choices

The following dishes originate from southern India and are excellent for the postnatal period. Choose from the following options.

non-vegetarian

All these dishes are served with boiled or steamed rice.

- Fish soup made with small fish.
- Dry fish shredded and fried or added as a garnish to cooked or sautéed vegetables.
- Chicken soup made with a whole small chicken.
- Chicken Roast made with butter, garlic and ginger (see recipe on page 128)

vegetarian options

- Vegetable soups made with vegetables of your choice. As a rule, throw in three different kinds of vegetable. Avoid broccoli, cauliflower and cabbage in the first six weeks as these may cause colic in the baby. Most other vegetables seem to be well tolerated.
- Drumstick leaves (available in Asian supermarkets), sautéed in sesame, coconut or sunflower oil.
- Garlic Curry (see recipe opposite).
- Buttermilk made into a light curry.
- Raagi kallie (postnatal pudding made from millet seeds, see recipe on page 35).
- Ommam kallie, made from lovage seeds/ajwain (see recipe on page 132).

Recipe for Ommam Kallie

Eat a quantity that corresponds to the size of a small lemon, twice a day.

100g of lovage seeds
100g of jaggery
200ml of sesame oil

1 Soak the lovage seeds for an hour, then make into a paste using a pestle and mortar. Do not use a food processor.
2 Mix with the other ingredients and cook on a low heat until the mixture can be rolled into a ball and rolls off the sides of the saucepan.
3 Let it cool and consume in small doses.

---

super saffron

Saffron is a digestive agent. Dissolve a few strands of saffron in half a cup of warm goat's milk and drink with a teaspoon of maple syrup. This is quite a treat!

---

exercise

Exercise for the new mother is an emotive and divisive issue. On the one hand, there are those who have neither the energy nor the inclination to start an exercise regime on top of everything else they're learning to deal with. On the other, there are those mothers who go for an ambitious walk two days after the birth, determined to prove they're 'back' and that their body is theirs once more.

Unfortunately, neither is the right approach. Although there's an overwhelming temptation to collapse on the sofa every time the baby snoozes (which you should do for the first three months), eventually your body's recovery will need a little more help from you. If you ever want to see your stomach muscles regain their former contours, then you've got to bring some light exercise into your life.

If you ever want to see your stomach muscles regain their former contours, then you've got to bring some light exercise into your life.

Note the word 'light'. It's an important qualification. After everything your body's been through, all it needs is some gentle activity to improve muscle tone. For as long as you're breastfeeding, the levels of the hormone relaxin (responsible for keeping your ligaments soft and bendy) remain as high as they did during pregnancy. This means your muscles and ligaments are not supporting your skeleton as securely as usual. Therefore all high-impact sports like running and skipping are out, and any stretching routine (pilates, yoga) must be followed conservatively.

Equally, if you embark on an ambitious exercise routine that saps you of calories, you risk exhausting yourself, and depleting your milk supply. As I discussed in 'How to Make Great Milk' (page 33), your body needs 500 extra calories a day to support your new milk supply.

The plus side – and yes, there is one – is that even light exercise will give you more energy than you had before. It will improve your muscle tone – making you look better – and restore your strength. It's crucial for you to have time away from your baby, and exercise provides a window of opportunity for you to focus on your mental and physical wellbeing. Appropriate exercise will assist your body's instinctive healing process and help to draw a line under your pregnant state.

pilates routine from six to twelve weeks

My Pilates teacher, Sandra Bickmore, advises mothers to commence exercise at six weeks, after a routine postnatal checkup with their midwife or doctor. This respects the fact that the mother's body needs time to recover from the birth. By six weeks the placental hormones, like relaxin, are at lower levels in her body, making exercising safer.

Here Sandra presents a series of eight easy and gentle postnatal Pilates exercises that you can safely follow at home. If you've got a Caesarean scar, be extra cautious and perform the moves smoothly. Avoid other sports and activities that might increase pressure on the abdomen, such as straining to hit a tennis ball.

PHYSICAL GOALS

- To correct overstretched abdominal muscles.
- To bring together split tummy muscles (divaricated rectus abdominus muscle).
- A desire to regain your pre-pregnant shape and have better overall muscle tone.

SOME QUESTIONS TO ASK YOURSELF BEFORE STARTING

- Do I have pelvic pain following the birth?
- Did I have pelvic pain before the birth?
- Do I feel instability in my pelvic joints?
- Does my pelvic floor feel weak (i.e. weak bladder neck)?
- Do I have a sagging feeling within the vagina?
- Do I have back pain?

If you answer yes to any of the first three questions, consult your GP before starting the routine. If you answer yes to any of the latter three, proceed gently and slowly.

the eight principles of the pilates method

1 Concentration
2 Breathing
3 Centring
4 Control (strength)
5 Precision
6 Flowing movement
7 Isolation in flexibility
8 Routlne

1 Relaxation Position

Aim: To prepare the mind and body for exercise. This position can also be used as a starting and finishing position for exercises. It releases unwanted tension from the body, allowing the torso to widen and the spine to lengthen.

Lic on a mat. Bend your knccs. Placc your fcct in linc with thc hips. Your second toe should be in line with the centre of the knee. Keep your feet parallel. Your neck should be released and lengthened, and you should feel comfortable.

Joseph Pilates: 'To breathe correctly you must completely exhale and inhale, always trying very hard to squeeze every atom of impure air from your lungs in much the same manner that you would wring every drop of water from a wet cloth.'

2 Breathing in the Relaxation Position

Aim: To combine lateral breathing with the relaxation position to encourage tension release and focus.

Lie in the Relaxation Position. Place your hands on your lower ribcage (Fig. 1). Breathe in wide and full into your sides, feeling the spine lengthen and open as you inhale.

Exhale – breathe out and allow the ribs to close together, taking the breath as low as you can into your pubic bone. Gently feel your lower abdominal muscles engage.

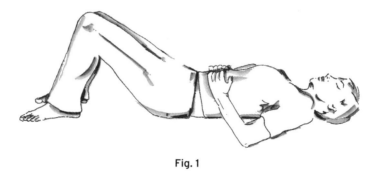

Fig. 1

Sensible exercise is beneficial to maintain the health of pregnant and postnatal mothers. It is absolutely vital to exercise at appropriate levels, taking it gently and building up a set of exercises to increase strength and mobility.

3 One-leg Lifts

Aim: Basic abdominal connection for the lower abdominal muscles.

Lie in the Relaxation Position. Breathing out, draw the right knee towards your chest without the right buttock lifting off the ground. Do not place any pressure on the floor with the left foot (Fig. 2).

As the foot is lifted off the floor, you may feel the abdominal muscles push up against your fingers. As you exhale, feel the abdominal muscles draw away from the fingers. Hold the leg towards you for the in-breath, then breathe out as the leg is slowly lowered to the floor.

Be aware: Sigh as you breathe out and flatten your ribcage into the floor.

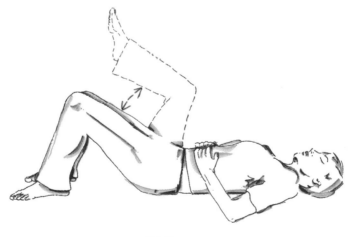

Fig. 2

4 Sliding Leg

Aim: Maintaining abdominal connection when the body is lengthening.

Lie on your back with legs extended and fingers placed on the lower abdominal muscles. Breathing out, bend one leg up to your chest, slowly sliding the foot along the floor to intensify control from the lower abdominal muscles (Fig. 3).

Breathe in as the leg slowly extends away, still drawing the abdominal muscles away from your fingers.

Be aware: Do not tighten the buttocks. On the breaths in and out, draw the ribs to the hips, breathing into the shoulder blades. Keep the neck lengthened and the shoulders relaxed. If the neck is arched, place a small cushion under the head.

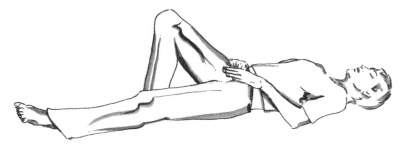

Fig. 3

5 The Starfish

Aim: To establish good movement and patterns throughout the body. So far we have been concentrating on the lower body. We also need to learn how to move the upper body whilst maintaining the neutral (starting) position and stability.

Start as in Sliding Leg. You are going to add the arms – if you slide up the right leg, the left arm goes over your head, so you are moving opposing limbs (Fig. 4). You may not be able to touch the floor comfortably so only move the arm as far as you can. Do not force the arm. The shoulder blade stays down into your back, and the ribs stay calm. Do not allow the back to arch at all.

Be aware: Imagine the abdominal muscles connected to the thigh, and that they are drawing in tighter as you bring the leg towards you. As the leg and arm extend away from you, let the abdominal muscles lengthen and flatten.

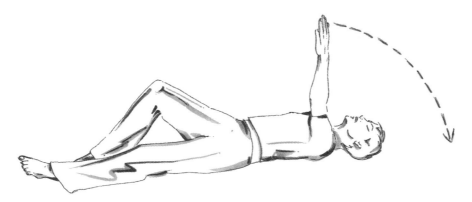

Fig. 4

6 Spine Curls with Pillow

Aim: To learn how to curl up the spine, vertebra by vertebra.
Equipment: Small cushion.

Lie in the Relaxation Position. Place the pillow between your knees. Your arms are relaxed by your side, palms down, fingers open.

Breathe in, preparing to lengthen the spine. Breathe out, centring. On the next in-breath, curl the spine away from the mat, vertebra by vertebra (Fig. 5). Inhale while you are raised, keeping the shoulders down and neck relaxed. As you exhale, imprint the spine slowly, starting from the chest and finishing with the tail bone.

Be aware: To lengthen the spine.

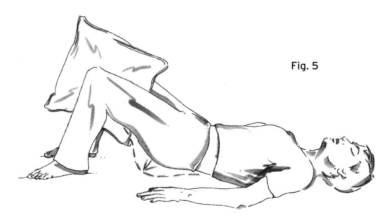

Fig. 5

7 The Star

Aim: To learn how to work from a strong, stable centre in your lower abdomen as you work the deep gluteal and upper-back muscles. (If you are uncomfortable lying on your stomach, place a small flat cushion under your abdomen to tilt the pelvis.)

Lie on your front, feet hip-width apart. Breathe in to prepare, and lengthen through the spine. Breathe out, taking the breath down into your pubic bone, feeling the lower abdominal muscles engage. Lift the left leg but not too high. Lengthen away from a strong centre, avoid tilting at the hips, and keep the bottom relaxed.

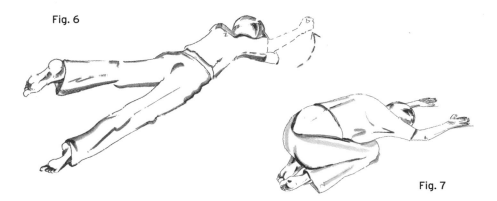

Fig. 6

Fig. 7

8 The Full Star

Start as for The Star, above. Then slide your arms out in front of you, keeping your shoulders away from the ears. Breathe in to prepare and lengthen through the spine. Breathe out, feeling the abdominal muscles engage, then lengthen and raise an arm and the opposite leg (Fig. 6). Breathe in and relax, then repeat on the other side.

When you have finished The Full Star, come up onto all fours and back into the Rest Position (Fig. 7).

pelvic floor exercises

The pelvic floor comprises three areas – the urethral, vaginal and anal muscles (situated in the front, middle and back of the pelvic floor). It is important to tone all three to restore full continence. Stress incontinence – urinary leaks when you cough or sneeze – is common postnatally, unless you have had an elective Caesarean.

Your pelvic floor muscles are exercised automatically when you perform Pilates-type exercises. The fascia covering the pelvic floor and the muscles of the abdominal wall are continuous so we do not have to target the pelvic floor to strengthen it. Every step you take automatically exercises your pelvic floor! However, for more specific control we need to be able to isolate and 'switch on' the key muscles in our lower abdomen; this automatically engages the pelvic floor and strengthens it appropriately.

In the first six weeks after birth, I tell my mothers to relax about the pelvic floor routine. Of course, it is very important to strengthen the pelvic floor area as soon as possible, but in the first month bruising and stretching means many mothers cannot feel the precise movements of their muscles down there! After six weeks or so, your pelvic tissues will feel as if they are coming back to normal and you can begin to focus on more specific exercises.

PELVIC FLOOR ROUTINE AT SIX WEEKS

To begin with, concentrate on tiny muscular movements. I advise squeezing the middle gluteal (buttock) and lower abdominal muscles, as much as possible and wherever you are – sitting in the car, eating lunch, lying on the sofa. It's important to remember that all the fascia (layers of skin, muscle and fat) are interconnected and that if you squeeze one, there is a waterfall effect which cascades down the layers. This is helpful in the early weeks because you can see, feel and control the large motor movement, and rest assured that it is gently toning on a smaller scale at the pelvic floor level.

PELVIC FLOOR ROUTINE AT EIGHT WEEKS

After eight weeks, concentrate on the urethral muscles at the front and squeeze in pulses for a count of three. On three, hold the squeeze and concentrate on drawing the contraction further up into your body. Hold and pulse for a count of three, then release. Repeat for the vaginal and anal muscles.

sleep

Sleep is to the new mother what birth is to the pregnant woman – the subject of apocryphal stories: how little sleep you get, how much your baby gets, the irony of post-natal insomnia. Everyone has a story about some aspect of post-partum sleep. What is certain is that with your baby's birth, sleep has become a commodity – something rare, precious and to be protected.

With your baby's birth, sleep has become a commodity – something rare, precious and to be protected.

newborn sleeping patterns

Newborn babies typically sleep for eighteen out of twenty-four hours. This sounds a lot until you break it down into a series of catnaps. As they grow, their tummies get proportionately bigger, allowing them to take bigger feeds and therefore sleep for longer periods. For you, this means three to four-hourly cycles of sleep, feed, change, play, sleep, before starting again. And so it repeats through the day and all through the night. Babies have no concept of night or day, only hunger, so the mother must bend to her baby's physical limitations in those initial weeks.

It's exhausting, of course it is, but it isn't forever. Successfully getting through this period and minimizing the stress it brings requires abandoning any notion of sleeping for more than four hours at a stretch in the first month, and instead napping, or at least resting, when the baby does. This is the very foundation of the red tent concept, and you should be vigilant in following it for the first three months. You are waking and sleeping just like your newborn baby. After twelve weeks, he's able to fit in with your more regulated cycle, and life will become more recognizable, but adapting to a new, temporary sleep pattern is just the first of the many changes you will readily make for your baby.

postnatal insomnia

It always makes my mothers roll their eyes when I give them a copy of my sleep tape at their postnatal session – after all, you're expecting to be dropping on your feet. Surely it's a case of selling ice to Eskimos? But actually – and ironically – postnatal insomnia is quite common and relates to high anxiety, be it anticipating the baby waking up or not being able to tune out the baby's every breath and snore! In most cases, the insomnia is resolved as the mother settles into her new role, acquires confidence in her maternal capabilities, and begins to trust that the baby himself is sleeping for longer and longer stretches. But extreme cases can require psychotherapy and/or hypnotherapy, and it's important that you do not wait too long before seeking professional help. Chronic exhaustion can contribute to postnatal depression, depleting your emotional and physical reserves, and can compromise your skills and confidence as a mother.

birth recovery: two to six weeks

- **Massage.** Continue with the rose otto massages – administered by your partner – for the first month (see page 46). From week five, you can do them yourself after your bath or shower each day. These massages are an important way of caring for yourself (very often overlooked when there's a gorgeous baby to compete with!) and will help alleviate any sad, detached or anxious feelings.
- **Aromatherapy.** Put a couple of drops of lavender or peppermint essential oil in your bath (avoid if you are taking any homeopathic remedies such as arnica). These oils have anti-inflammatory properties, and are relaxants for the muscles and central nervous system.
- **If your baby is windy,** eliminate caffeine and alcohol, and drink fennel or nettle tea.
- **Birth acceptance.** If you haven't already done so, write down or discuss your birth story with your partner, midwife or obstetrician, and get answers to all your questions, no matter how small or niggling they might seem. Address this whilst the experience is still fresh in everyone's mind so that you can fully accept your baby's birth and move on (see page 50).
- **Creative healing treatments.** See a qualified practitioner for another female treatment, or ask your partner to perform some bladder and pelvic drainage (see Resources for DVD to do at home).
- **Muscle release.** Ask your partner to gently perform some massage on your shoulders, neck and upper back. This can be done with oils. Even as your muscles recover from the birth, you will be tiring these areas by holding the baby for long periods and breastfeeding, so it is important to keep them soft, clear and relaxed.
- **Cranio-sacral therapy.** I advise seeing a therapist to dissipate any residual fascial and intra-cranial tension from the birth.

- **Reflexology.** Regular reflexology on your hands and/or feet will help boost kidney function and assist the elimination of body fluids after the birth.
- **Pelvic floor routine.** In a lying position, with knees bent and feet flat on the floor, lift your buttocks a few inches off the floor and tip your pubic bone up as if curling round to your belly button. Pull your tummy in, hold for five and release. Repeat five times.
- **Catnaps.** Continue to catnap when your baby sleeps. You should be having at least one two- to three-hour sleep during the day.
- **Walking.** Go for daily walks with the baby, if the weather allows. This will help boost lymphatic drainage, bring back some muscular strength and tone, and introduce some mild fat burning.
- **Visitors.** Begin to accept some visitors, or go out on social visits. Having a couple of hours of social time once or twice a week will help bring some normality back into your life, and reduce the isolating 'twilight zone' effect.

pregnancy recovery: seven to twelve weeks

- **Pilates.** An ideal form of exercise, as described above.
- **Light exercise.** Introduce a light exercise routine such as walking, cycling, rowing or swimming (if you are sure your perineum has healed and your lochia has stopped). In the first twelve weeks avoid strenuous sports like tennis, running, skipping, skiing, riding and skating!
- **Massage.** Perform a pre-shower Ayurvedic warm oil massage with cured sesame oil or postnatal Ayurvedic oil. After a shower or bath use rose otto oil for a self-massage (see page 46).
- **Creative healing treatments.** See a practitioner for a digestive tune-up, spleen treatment (to restore blood count), back treatment (to help the ligaments slowly go back to their pre-pregnant shape), tummy toning and pelvic lift.

- **Bowen/cranio-sacral treatment.** I advise a Bowen and/or a cranio-sacral treatment at regular intervals from four weeks. This will deeply relax you and help rebalance your pelvis (the baby lies to one side or the other).
- **Refine your pelvic floor routine.** You should be able to feel smaller, more precise movements by now, and your previous exercises will have helped restore some muscle tone. Visualize the three areas of the pelvic floor – urethral at the front; vaginal in the middle; and anal at the back. Isolate each one and focus on contracting and pulsing each area separately, without moving any of the larger surrounding muscles (see page 143). Repeat 10 squeezes per area.
- **Sleep when your baby does.** By now you should be getting at least one sleep of five or more hours. Express some milk and ask your partner to do one of the night feeds so that you can sleep for a longer stretch.
- **Sex.** At your six-week postnatal check, you will ideally be examined to see if you have any tender areas in your vagina. If all is well you are free to resume sexual relations with your partner. This time frame allows for the lochia to stop, your vagina to heal and any bruising to subside. However, it is very much a guideline, and if it still feels too early for penetration, then rest assured that most other people feel exactly the same way as you (see page 179). You may need to use a lubricating agent such as KY Jelly in the beginning until your hormone levels restore your natural moisture.
- **Take Ashwagandha (*Withania somnifera*).** This is a well-researched, anti-stress herb that I advise both parents to take from four to six weeks after the birth when you may begin to feel run down. It has been studied extensively and been found to nurture the nervous system and counteract anxiety (ideal for treating postnatal depression). It has anti-inflammatory properties and is easily the most potent aphrodisiac in the entire botanical kingdom! Solgar sell it in capsule form. The dosage for both partners is one capsule twice a day for as long as you need the boost. It is quite safe for breastfeeding mothers.

- **Take Gotu-Kola tincture.** This is available on the shelf in most health-food stores. Thirty drops a day in water serves as a powerful immuno-modulant for men and women. It addresses common symptoms such as tiredness, insomnia and stress – making it an ideal postnatal herb – as well as speeding up wound healing and reducing scar tissue formation.

treatment summary for practitioners and partners

You can follow the instructions on my DVD for creative healing and reflexology (see Resources).

WEEK TWO
Creative Healing (must do!)

- General lymphatic treatment and a full back and neck treatment.
- Abdominal toning and pelvic drainage (only if you have had a vaginal delivery). For Caesarean sections, all abdominal treatments are performed about 3 to 4 inches off the surface of the body as we stroke the aura, and the effects are felt in the underlying tissues.
- Heart treatment.
- Kidney treatment.

Reflexology (must do!)

General relaxation and drainage treatment. Specific areas to work on include the pituitary gland and hypothalamus, kidney points, back and neck areas and the lymphatic reflexes. The aim is to help eliminate extra-cellular fluid from the body.

Cranio-sacral Treatment

The mother's and baby's cranio-sacral system will have been challenged by the stresses and strains of delivery. An appropriate treatment will realign tissues that might have been stretched during labour and restore function.

Bowen Technique

Has very similar benefits to cranial therapy. I find it extremely useful at all times during pregnancy and the postnatal phase. Specific moves: the breast moves, performed in an elliptical fashion around each breast. These can relieve breast engorgement and prevent mastitis (see page 292).

Self-hypnosis and Visualization

Practise deep muscle relaxation and self-hypnosis to promote self-healing and deep sleep. I have a postnatal toning-up CD that can help your body return to its pre-pregnant levels and be even more beautiful than before! (See Resources.)

Colour/light Therapy (for mother and baby)

Three treatments a week for three weeks can reduce the effect of prenatal and birth trauma. These can be started as early as possible after the birth.

Creative Healing (must do!)

- General treatment and full back treatment.
- Abdominal toning and pelvic drainage.
- Full digestive tune-up, including the pancreatic treatment and liver drainage.
- A spleen treatment to replenish your blood constituents, such as red blood cells, white blood cells and the lymphocytes.
- Female treatment.

Reflexology (must do!)

Weekly reflexology gives the mother much-needed relaxation. The mother has to spend hours getting up at night and this can cause disrupted sleep. Reflexology is very good at promoting deep sleep, even though you can only sleep in short bursts!

Cranio-sacral Treatment

Please try and schedule one. You may only need to see the cranial therapist once every two to four weeks.

Bowen Technique

As in week two, the breast moves can relieve engorgement and prevent mastitis.

Creative Healing (must do!)

Perform the following treatments for general toning, helping to ease the neck and back and balance out muscle tension that might be caused by breastfeeding:

- General treatment.
- Back and neck treatment.
- Abdominal toning – helps the tummy muscles go back to their pre-pregnant shape, size and tone.

Reflexology (must do)

Professional reflexology is advised on a weekly basis or use my reflexology DVD and get your partner or a friend to watch the DVD and perform the moves. This way you will be able to keep up the treatments.

You need an all-round reflexology treatment. It's important to work on the breast lymphatics to keep the breast milk flowing and to prevent congestion. By now you can work gently on the uterine reflex areas and help them to eliminate any final threads of lochia. Stimulating the hypothalamus and pituitary gland areas will be very useful to keep up the hormones of lactation, namely oxytocin and prolactin.

Bowen Technique

It's good to continue a series of six Bowen treatments to help you relax deeply and to strengthen the back muscles and ligaments as they slowly release the effects of relaxin and go back to their pre-pregnant tone. Your Bowen practitioner will teach you to perform the breast moves in an elliptical fashion around each breast. These can relieve engorgement and prevent mastitis.

Cranio-sacral Treatment

If you have already seen a cranial therapist, you will probably have been asked to come back every two to four weeks for follow-up treatments. Do take a friend along to baby-sit while you are receiving a treatment. You and your practitioner will agree how often you and your baby need to attend for sessions.

WEEK FIVE
Creative Healing (must do!)

- Back and neck drainage: twenty minutes.
- Abdominal toning: ten minutes.

Reflexology (must do!)

An all-round deep treatment to tone and revitalize.

Bowen Technique

If you have embarked on a series of Bowen treatments, it is advisable to complete six in a row.

Homeopathic Consultation

See a homeopath to discuss constitutional remedies for both mother and baby, and to discuss immunization issues.

WEEK SIX
Creative Healing (must do!)

- General treatment.
- Abdominal toning: for ten minutes as a prelude to the female treatment and the pelvic organ lift. This repositions the cervix and the bladder neck in the pre-pregnant position within the pelvis and prevent all degrees of uterine and bladder neck prolapse. For instance, the pelvic lift can correct retroversion of the uterus quite easily – I have verified this by performing pelvic examinations before and after the pelvic lift.
- A full digestive tune-up could be given every three weeks.

Reflexology (must do!)

If any single treatment can make you feel rejuvenated it is reflexology. It acts as a detox and mental booster as well as a colon regulator.

WEEK SEVEN
Creative Healing

- Weekly general treatments will keep your back and neck mobile.

Reflexology

Continue weekly reflexology sessions.

WEEK EIGHT
Creative Healing

- Weekly general treatments will keep your back and neck mobile.
- Heart treatment once every four weeks.

Reflexology

Continue general all-round weekly reflexology sessions.

Cranio-sacral Treatment

Have your four-weekly top-up.

Reflexology

Continue weekly reflexology sessions.

Creative Healing

- Weekly general treatments will keep your back and neck mobile.
- Full digestive tune-up every three weeks.

Reflexology

Continue weekly reflexology sessions.

Creative Healing

- Weekly general treatments will keep your back and neck mobile.

Reflexology

Continue weekly reflexology sessions.

Creative Healing

- Weekly general treatments will keep your back and neck mobile.
- Abdominal treatment and a female treatment.

Reflexology

Continue weekly reflexology sessions.

Creative Healing

- General treatment and back and neck treatments will keep your back and neck mobile.
- Heart treatment.

Cranio-sacral Treatment

Have your four-weekly treatments.

PART TWO
discovery

three to six months

baby

Congratulations! You're through the worst and are now entering what is considered to be the golden age of babyhood. Your baby will be crying much less (and if she's suffered from colic, life will become dramatically better). She should be rounding out and looking rosy, and be fascinated by her environment. Here's what you can expect.

sleep

The development that will probably make most difference to your days is your baby's night. By now, she should be sleeping for at least an eight- to ten-hour stretch, and most babies are capable of sleeping for a full twelve-hour period. If your baby is still only 'napping' for a few hours at night, it's really important to check she's not sleeping too much in the day, and to bring in a regulated sleeping routine as soon as possible. Chronic overtiredness will impair her concentration and growth, and lead to grumpiness and hyperactive behaviour.

By now, your baby should be sleeping for at least an eight- to ten-hour stretch, and most babies are capable of sleeping for a full twelve-hour period.

Some mothers think their baby sleeps less, and often say 'She's always so alert/overexcited' – but these are classic symptoms of overtiredness, and you'll be amazed at how much your baby begins to sleep once she gets into the groove. Sleep is vital to our health, and the newborn's body instinctively 'shuts down' into sleep when it has assimilated enough stimulus. But by three months, once she's adapted to her new environment, this instinct is fading. Sleep becomes less automatic and more of a habitual need, as the body relies on bigger sleeps being supplied at longer, but fixed, intervals.

daytime naps

By three to six months, your baby will need only up to three hours' sleep in the day. Most mothers follow one of two options: either two biggish sleeps in the day (ninety minutes mid-morning; ninety minutes mid-afternoon) or two thirty-minute naps (mid-morning and mid-afternoon) punctuated by a big sleep over the lunchtime period (ninety minutes to two hours).

Deciding which option to take really boils down to how you like to run your day – some mothers like to organize activities in the mornings and afternoons and enjoy some quiet time at home over the lunch period. Other mothers like to have quieter mornings and afternoons focused around a more sociable out-and-about lunchtime. Whichever way you work it, there should be at least two spells in the day spent quietly at home. As I mentioned in the previous chapter, I do think it's important to put the baby to sleep in her cot, as regardless of when you take it, your own rest should coincide with hers. This does restrict your movements somewhat but it will give you a vital recharging period (post-red tent), and most mothers come to guard this precious time jealously.

physical independence

Distance and time will take on different meanings to you in this period because you'll suddenly get a bit more of both. By now, your baby probably loves nothing more than lying under her baby gym – kicking, wriggling and hitting the toys – and as she spends longer and longer periods amusing herself, you will be able to move more freely, including out of eyeshot.

The mechanics of running a family and household become so much easier when you don't have to carry a baby about with you constantly. And even when you do have the baby with you: look – one hand! Head control is usually mastered by four months so you can now begin to carry your baby about safely on your hip – it's such a small gesture, but brings with it so much more freedom. Colic or windiness also dissipate with head control as the muscular strength required to support the head coincides with digestive maturity. And, tantalizingly, your baby is getting her first glimpses of an upright world. This is a major change of perspective, which delights and puzzles her, and from now on, she'll be rolling and wriggling her way to independent sitting.

becoming mobile

You can easily trace and predict the path of your baby's growing mobility, because everything starts with the head and works gradually down the body, moving from the gross motor skills to the fine motor skills. So, for instance, once head control has been mastered, your baby will gain control of the arms (swiping), hands (grabbing) and finally fingers (picking up). Once the arms are under control, legs are next, moving from kicking to rolling (to some frantic toe-chewing), crawling, cruising and finally stepping. Of course, these developmental milestones overlap each other and occur over an eighteen-month period. But knowing roughly what to expect can help you encourage and foster the next stage.

playtime

You'll find that your baby's growing physical independence will redefine how you play together. Head control means the advent of (gentle) rough and tumble, baby gymnastics (bringing her feet to her mouth for example) and interactive games. Your baby will love it when you act out the following nursery rhymes with her:

INTERACTIVE RHYMING GAMES

Row, Row, Row Your Boat

Row, row, row your boat
Gently down the stream
Merrily, merrily, merrily, merrily
Life is but a dream.

(sit facing each other holding hands, gently push and pull backwards and forwards)

Rock, rock, rock your boat
Gently to and fro
Merrily, merrily, merrily, merrily
Down the stream we go.

(sit facing each other holding hands, making small side rocks)

Row, row, row your boat
Gently down the stream
And if you see a crocodile
Don't forget to scream.

(repeat movements as first verse)

(wave arms in air, little screams)

A variation on this game is lying on the floor with your knees bent and the baby sitting on your tummy. Holding the baby's hands, gently and slowly lower her as you roll up to a sitting position, and bring the baby up again as you roll back down – like a seesaw motion. It's also good tummy exercise for you!

Fiddledy Diddledy Dee

Fiddledy diddledy dee   *(knees bent, baby sitting on top)*
Bounce you on my knee
Fiddledy diddledy dough   *(straighten legs out, gently lay*
Drop you down a hole – whee!   *baby flat)*
Fiddledy diddledy di
Lift you way up high   *(lift baby above your face)*
Fiddledy diddledy do
I love you   *(cuddle close)*

Zoom, Zoom, Zoom

Zoom, zoom, zoom   *(baby sitting in your lap)*
We're going to the moon.
Zoom, zoom, zoom
We'll be there very soon.
5, 4, 3, 2, 1 – blast off!   *(lift baby high into the air)*

This is the Way the Ladies Ride

This is the way the ladies ride   *(sit on chair; baby facing you, on*
Trittetty trot, trittetty trot   *your knee)*
This is the way the ladies ride
Trittetty, trittetty trot.   *(little, fast bumps)*

This is the way the gentlemen ride
Gallopy-trot, gallopy-trot   *(bigger, slower bumps)*
This is the way the gentlemen ride
Gallopy, gallopy, trot.

This is the way the farmers ride
Hobbledy hoi, hobbledy hoi   *(lurching, deep bumps)*
This is the way the farmers ride
Hobbledy, hobbledy, hoi
And – down – into the ditch!   *(push feet out, legs straight, let*
     baby lie back as though fallen)

teething

One thing that will rock the boat during these calm waters is teething. It can come on any time from twelve weeks (although some babies cut a tooth a little before that) and start as late as one year, but the average age of the onset of teething is between four and five months.

The teeth you can expect to greet first are the lower central pair, followed by the two upper central teeth. Once they begin to come through, they usually pop up in pairs or small clusters within a week or so of each other. However, getting there can sometimes be a long wait. For six to eight weeks you might be constantly attributing her grumpy behaviour to teething, without any evidence whatsoever to back you up. The hallmarks of teething are:

- red cheeks
- fever
- nappy rash
- excessive drooling
- discomfort sucking on the bottle
- biting down
- irritability
- disturbed sleep

These are difficult to go through, and you may well wonder whether this is actually just your baby's true personality finally shining forth. But have faith. A shiny pearl will emerge from those red gums and happiness will be quickly restored.

Teething will continue on and off until roughly the age of three, when all the milk teeth are in (until the age of six to seven when you have to start all over again). You will become accustomed to the change in your baby's behaviour, but there is a lot you can do to soothe your baby during the worst periods:

- Treat the fever (with your doctor's permission) with infant paracetamol.
- Nelson's offer a specific homeopathic teething remedy called Teetha, which is particularly useful for the first few teeth (molars and canines usually need a bit more help).
- Refrigerated carrot or cucumber sticks soothe hot little gums and will taste softly pleasant to your baby too.
- Most good pharmacists stock gel- or water filled teething toys, which can be kept cool in the fridge (but never in the freezer, which can cause ice burns).
- Wooden rattles are great for biting down on.
- Change dirty nappies immediately as they tend to be more acidic during teething, which can really irritate the baby's skin.
- Stick to a good organic nappy cream, like Weleda's, during teething episodes. If your baby's bottom becomes particularly excoriated, move up to a stronger nappy cream such as Metanium or Sudocream.
- Make sure your baby is getting plenty of rest, especially if she is being disturbed by the pain during the night. Allow ten minutes extra per nap, more if necessary, depending upon the length of the night wakings.

Another thing to be aware of is that bad teething episodes can coincide with short illnesses, suggesting that teething can lower the baby's immune system and make her more susceptible to colds and bugs. So try to boost your baby's natural reserves with a constitutional homeopathic remedy that can be prescribed by a homeopath (see Resources).

dental routine

Once the teeth are through and the gum inflammation has subsided, you can begin a mild dental routine. Many of the premium dental brands have specially-designed first toothbrushes that are extra-soft to prevent abrasion on tender gums. You should also use only specially formulated baby homeopathic toothpastes, as adult versions have too much fluoride. Only a tiny amount (petit pois size) needs to be squeezed onto the brush.

---
note

Antibiotics can occasionally cause a reaction in your baby's saliva that coats the teeth with a sticky plaque. Be extra vigilant with brushing if your baby has to take a course of antibiotics for any reason.

- If your baby is teething very young, a toothbrush may feel very large for her mouth. Try using a soft-bristled small fingertip brush instead.
- If your baby hates the feel of the bristles full-stop, squeeze a blob of toothpaste onto a clean flannel and drape it over your index finger. Use your finger as the brush for the first few weeks, occasionally interspersing with a real toothbrush until she accepts it.
- When you move on to beakers and cups, avoid the non-spill variety. They are fitted with anti-leak valves which force the baby to suck extra hard to extract the drink. More and more dentists are reporting problems with babies and infants who have damaged their jaws with this vigorous sucking. Either remove the valve from the non-leak beakers (which, remember, will mean the cup's contents can spill) or look for specially-designed easy-flow cups.
- When you begin to offer drinks other than milk (once your baby start solids), offer water and avoid fruit juice altogether – milk teeth have weaker enamel which is more easily corroded by sugars. Your baby has no comprehension of what juice is, so she has absolutely no need of it.
- You do not need to take your baby for a dental checkup until she is around two years old.
- If thumb-sucking or dummies are being used as constant soothers, do try switching to an orthodontic dummy and consult your dentist.

For the first few attempts at brushing, your baby may recoil from the unfamiliar taste so just let her grab the brush between her teeth whilst she gets used to the flavour and explores the bristles with her tongue. After a week or so of this, she will be used to the taste and feel, and will be more inclined to let you gently brush the teeth. You may only get 20 seconds of brushing done but try to increase that each week. Two minutes is what you should be aiming for by two years of age.

baby care

- From three months, your baby will prefer to be propped up more, rather than lying flat on her back. Either do this with some cushions, or invest in an inflatable 'nest' which allows the baby to see more of what's going on and keeps her safely enclosed, preventing her from falling forwards or to the side, or needing to be protected from marauding older siblings.
- If you have a baby backpack, your baby will love sitting in this now and being taken on walks by you or her father.
- From three months, put a few drops of aromatherapy oil, such as lavender, in the bath.
- Your baby is beginning to grasp object permanence – that an object continues to exist, even if she cannot see it. Games like peek-a-boo reinforce this. Hide your face behind your hands, drape a piece of muslin over your baby's head or cover a favourite toy with a towel. Give your baby a minute or so to react – she will soon begin to pull off the towel and expect to see the toy still there.
- At three months, your baby's eyesight is vastly improved and she will begin to track moving objects. Swing a pendulum, walk your fingers up and down her legs or move a pull-along toy across the floor.
- Hearing has developed to the point where your baby is now filtering out unnecessary stimulus of background or 'white' noise, and focuses on sounds that are important or interesting. Your baby will quickly turn towards your voice now (even though your voice is already a familiar sound, long before this stage), so speak to her from across the room and encourage her to detect and locate sound.
- If you have kept up your baby's tummy mat work (see page 103), she will by now be strong enough to begin to roll onto her back regularly

(make sure she is lying on a soft blanket or rug, as she may still drop her head down and bang it on the floor at the beginning). It'll be a few more weeks before she rolls from her back onto her tummy as her head is relatively heavy and so requires a lot more tummy strength and a strong neck.

- If your baby has a favourite physical habit – such as rotating her ankles, or becoming as 'stiff as a board' when you try to get her pyjamas on – be sure to name it and repeat it every time you notice her doing this. She will soon learn to perform the action if you just name it, which is an early instance of playing to the crowd, and is both charming to you and exciting to her.
- Your baby will be using smiles, laughs and gurgles to communicate now, instead of so much crying.
- At four months, your baby will begin to coo. I call this the 'love dove' stage. Coo back to her and try to mimic her own timings and inflections. Believe it or not, this is the first step towards speech.
- Build up your repertoire of daily sing-songs as they are also important in speech development.
- Encourage physical activity by holding your baby firmly around the waist and getting her to do little jumps up and down on a soft rug. This will help develop leg strength and get her ready for crawling.
- Your baby is naturally flexible and will only lose it if it is not used. When she starts reaching for her toes – which seem very exotic to her – and trying to nibble them, give a little helping hand to the flexing action. Your little yogi will enjoy the gentle stretch.
- Your baby has a good grasp by now and will be actively reaching out and swiping at things (developing hand-eye co-ordination and spatial perception).
- Your baby is learning about texture by placing everything in her mouth. This is known as mouthing. Make sure she has a variety of surfaces to play with – smooth hard plastic, hollow wood, soft knobbly rubber, Velcro, knits or crochet, plush velour … (Note: make sure all objects are large and cannot be completely put into

the mouth so there is no risk of choking. Choose objects that do not shed fibres or have small parts that can be broken off.)

- Adapt the Tiger in the Tree position (previously used as a calming hold, page 77) to become a flying aeroplane. Lay your baby on your forearm with your hand beneath her tummy and grabbing the opposite armpit, and with your second hand between the legs, grasping a thigh. Gently and very, very slowly, 'fly' her through the air to your partner. Your baby will love being suspended and swayed, the feeling of the air flowing over her face, seeing the world from up high and rushing excitingly to daddy!

- Give your baby soft cloth books to mouth, explore and practise turning pages. Your baby will now also be able to cope with more complex pictures and images in secondary, blended colours (such as purple, green, pink and brown) and with more background detail.

- Your baby will not yet 'fill' her car seat. When you're travelling on longer journeys you may notice that her head lolls to the side at an awkward angle when she sleeps. So take an old pashmina or other tasselled scarf of yours (so that it smells of you) and fold it in half lengthways. Wrap it around your baby's neck and bring the tasselled end loosely through the loop in the middle. This will do many things: keep your baby warm; your baby's fingers will love playing with the tassles; it will support her head more comfortably; and of course it will smell of you and so comfort your baby.

- To encourage rolling and tummy shuffling, place a few toys to your baby's side just out of reach. Let her try to get them on her own for a few minutes, but then push them nearer within reach, otherwise she will become frustrated and give up.

massage routine

After twelve weeks, you can add an aromatherapy element. The smells are potent, however, so check your baby likes the aroma before covering her in it. Try adding to 15ml of base oil or sweet almond oil one of the following options:

- one drop of lavender oil, ideal for inducing sleepiness
- one drop of camomile roman, soothing for fractious babies
- one drop of tea tree oil, a good constitutional tonic
- one drop of rose otto or sweet violet, ideal for babies prone to dry skin conditions such as eczema
- one drop of eucalyptus oil, good when your baby has a cold and lots of mucus

Note: Remember some aromatherapy oils such as rosemary, tea tree or eucalyptus reduce the potency of homeopathy treatments. Floral oils are generally okay.

---

tip

If the aromatherapy oils are not blending well with the base oil (ratio one drop of essential oil to 15ml of base oil) mix in a splash of milk. This helps the aromatherapy oil 'drop' into the base oil.

Before you lay your hands on the baby, hold up the palms of your hands and show them to her. She will come to recognize this gesture as the beginning of the massage routine.

With the baby lying on her back, perform long, light, sweeping strokes from her head down to her feet, lightly – you're just making her consciously aware of her body. Repeat fifteen times.

FACE

Place both your thumbs on her 'third eye' – the space between her eyebrows – and gently stroke outwards along the upper eyebrow line (Fig. 1). Repeat five times. With your thumbs, and the lightest of touches, trace small circles on her temples (Fig. 2). After five circles on the temples, rotate the circles down to the cheekbones and out to the ears. Take the ears between your bent fingers and thumbs and gently squeeze down to the earlobes. Very gently, pull the earlobes down a couple of times.

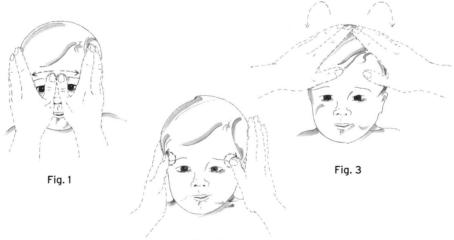

Fig. 1

Fig. 2

Fig. 3

HEAD

The head can be massaged ever so gently with tiny circular movements. First you move around the periphery of the scalp for one or two minutes. Then draw your hands almost off the scalp from the hairline above the forehead, over and above the top of the head down to the nape of the neck, just three or four times (Fig. 3).

Open your palms and lay your hands over the width of the baby's head, avoiding her face. You can let the baby feel the weight of your hands but still aim for a light touch. Gently run your hands over her head and ears, as though smoothing down her hair. Repeat rhythmically and lovingly for ten strokes. Remember to maintain eye contact.

SHOULDERS AND TORSO

After the last stroke, bring your hands to rest on the baby's shoulders. Press down very gently so that the shoulders relax beneath the partial weight of your hands. Place your right hand on the baby's right shoulder (Fig. 4) and sweep it down to her left hipbone. Repeat on the other side. Repeat the pattern so that your hands criss-cross rhythmically and continuously over the torso. This helps the baby feel centred and to join up all the different areas of her body. Repeat ten times. Finish with both hands on the lower tummy.

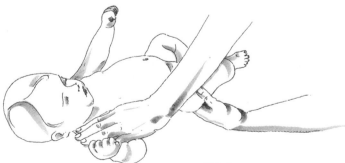

Fig. 4

Fig. 5   Fig. 6

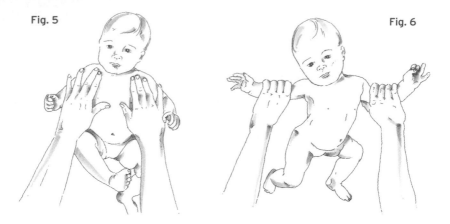

Keep both your hands on the centre of her tummy, with your fingers facing towards her head. Sweep up the centre of the torso, and fan out your fingers as you get to the shoulders so that your hands dip down over the shoulders towards the back (Fig. 5). Gently squeeze the large trapezius muscle before gliding your hands back over the shoulders and all the way down the arms (Fig. 6). Gently squeeze the palm of the baby's hand and then return your hands to her torso and repeat ten times. Finish with your hands on the centre of her tummy.

TUMMY

Rhythmically walk your middle three fingers from the lowest part of the abdomen up towards the ribcage (Fig. 7). This gets the baby used to the tummy – a very vulnerable area – being touched. You may find that your baby tenses the tummy initially but this is a natural guarding response. With practice, the baby begins to trust your touch, and after the first few sessions, she will relax into your tummy massage. Repeat for a minute.

Lay your hands side by side on one side of the baby's waist, fingers facing down to the ground. Briskly alternate gently pulling up the baby's waist and in towards the stomach for a couple of minutes. Repeat on the other side. This creates a lovely girdled 'held' feeling.

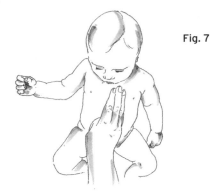

Fig. 7

Unlike other massage routines, the creative healing massage avoids going round and round the tummy, so the tummy section of the massage routine need last only one to two minutes.

ARMS AND HANDS

Massage one arm at a time, gently grasping the whole arm with your cupped hand. Use a generous quantity of oil so that your hand glides smoothly down the entire length of the arm from the armpit all the way down to the hands (Fig. 8).

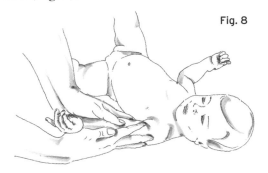

Fig. 8

Alternate your strokes between the right and left arms so that your baby can sense a rhythm in your massage. Then take each tiny hand and slowly define each finger by stroking and stretching it out gently, one by one. Hold each palm with the fingertips of both your hands and gently fan out your fingers and relax your baby's palm. A sort of hand reflexology massage!

Softly rotate your baby's hand at the wrist a few times, both clockwise and anticlockwise.

Gently take the baby's hands between your index fingers and thumbs. Softly do little pulsing squeezes around the palm area (not over the knuckles). Repeat for one minute.

LEGS AND FEET

Curl both your hands around the top of your baby's hip, one side at a time. Gently slide your hands down the front and the back of your baby's thigh and leg, taking care to slide the fingers lightly around, but not directly over, the knee (Fig. 9). Finish with a gentle squeeze of the foot and repeat ten times. Repeat on the other thigh and leg. The baby's instinct will be to curl the leg in, so gently uncurl the leg and keep it long and soft. Do not tug or jerk the leg. If the baby resists uncurling at all, just run your hands over the bent leg for the first few sessions.

Holding the baby's feet, gently push both legs back so that the baby bends her legs towards her stomach (like reverse abdominal curls). Repeat five times.

Gentleness is paramount for this next manoeuvre. Take the baby's thigh in one hand and the calf of the same leg in the other. Incredibly gently and slowly, squeeze the calf and thigh muscles in opposing directions. Avoid twisting the legs. This is a surface movement. Keep pressure off the knee at all times.

Then let one of your baby's feet rest in the cup of your hand as you gently massage small circles around the ankle bone for about a minute.

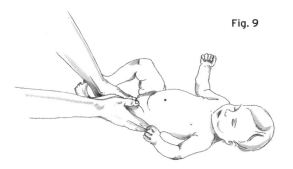

Fig. 9

Repeat this for about thirty seconds. This is the area of pelvic lymphatics in reflexology terms, so you are getting your baby off to a good start by establishing efficient lymphatic drainage channels.

Draw long strokes over the tops of the baby's foot, moving from heel to toes. Then with the pad of your thumb, gently press long lines up the soles of the baby's foot, finishing at the toes. Repeat for twenty seconds.

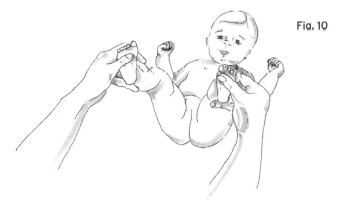

Fig. 10

Flex and point the baby's foot several times. Very, very gently, take each tiny toe and pass it through your fingers. Avoid twisting the toes. The movements are minute (Fig. 10).

Repeat this entire sequence on the other leg. Finish by holding both of the baby's feet in your hands. Gently shake out the legs, which should be really relaxed and floppy. With your thumbs, pulse a few squeezes into the soles of your baby's feet to finish.

BACK MASSAGE

If your baby is amenable to being placed on her tummy, turn her over with her arms outstretched for balance (she'll probably try to keep her head up for a bit). Gently walk your fingertips up each side of her spine lightly. Pressure can be reasonably firm.

Sweep your hands smoothly and confidently up the expanse of her back, fanning out at the shoulders (Fig. 11). Finish with a little squeeze at the top of the shoulder. Repeat several times.

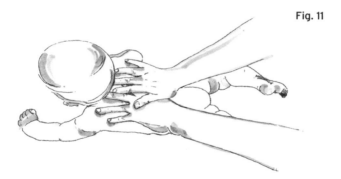

Fig. 11

Criss-cross your hands from one shoulder to opposite hip and repeat on the other side. Repeat ten times.

Finally, make a fist and gently make twisting motions with the flats of your fingers. Pressure should still be light. Work from the back of the hips up the body (again, avoiding direct contact on the spine).

Finish with a few light sweeping strokes from the top of the head to the toes.

mother

This period marks your emergence from the post-partum cocoon. You
will hopefully have had some secluded time as advocated by the historic
red tent, and I hope you will have rested, recovered and been restored
from the pregnancy and birth. Still, even with the most supported
confinement, this can be a tricky stage. Your baby is growing, and many
mothers feel there's an unspoken pressure to 'get on with it' – you may feel
that you would like to have your figure back and resume sexual relations.
How you actually feel and what you may think you are supposed to feel
can be poles apart, but in my experience, this is usually a confidence lag.
It is in this short stage that the new family unit really settles down, life
takes on a more recognizable face at last, and the fun bit finally begins!

sexual relationships

The biggest of all these 'business as usual' worries has to be post-baby
sex. Women are very shy about discussing this subject – it is almost
taboo – and yet worries, fear and dissatisfaction surrounding it are
practically universal. Very few people slip back into their old bedroom
habits without some mini crisis.

I have deliberately included this topic here, rather than in the previous
chapter, because six weeks is considered the earliest for couples to
resume their sexual relationship. But actually, most couples take their
first tentative steps back to each other during the second and third
months. It's usually a couple of weeks after that – when there is an
unspoken expectation for sex to become regular again – that underlying
issues begin to surface.

Once upon a time in your relationship, sex was the fun, passionate and
easy way for you and your partner to show how much you loved each

other. Then, when you were pregnant, it became something miraculous, giving and tender. Now, after your baby's birth, it may well feel alien, demanding, even a little frightening.

I get many mothers coming to me who, after long days of cuddling, kissing, stroking, dressing, bathing, feeding and changing their babies, feel quite literally 'touched out' by the evening. They feel conflicting emotions because of course they love to touch their babies, but it can come at a cost to their partner when they lose the energy or inclination to snuggle up on the sofa or share a kiss in the kitchen. When this is the case, dialogue between the parents is absolutely key because where there's exhaustion for one parent, there'll be frustration for the other.

reigniting the spark

Both parents may feel that their needs deserve to be met at this time, but sometimes just articulating their frustration and knowing their partner has heard it can help dissipate the problem. Sexual harmony rarely happens if one partner feels pressured or rushed to resume full sex. That just leads to resentment. So, in the early weeks, the emphasis may well have to shift away from full sex, and move more towards flirtation and loving touch, keeping the sexual element there, but gently simmering on the back burner for a bit longer. Massage and bathing together are intrinsically relaxing and restoring, and both parents benefit from the intimacy they garner. Equally, little gestures like holding hands or giving lingering kisses 'hello' and 'goodbye' can reignite a spark.

The threat to many new parents is that in becoming a family, they cease to be a couple. All the intimate gestures, in-jokes, pet names and so on can be quickly forgotten when the very serious business of having a baby intrudes. For the mother particularly, her sense of identity will have been completely overhauled, and it's a rare woman who emerges from the mothering chrysalis the same as she went in. She's seen her body swell and subside; she's felt kicking from within and suckling from without; where she once shared her body with her partner, she is now 'outsourcing' it to a ravenous little babe.

There are several escape routes from this – very common – scenario, but all of them are underlined by time. Time really is the sexual healer. In time, your baby will start to sleep more and you'll feel less exhausted. In time, your baby will be weaned and your body will be yours again. In time, you'll get your figure back, and with it your sexual confidence. In time, your hormone levels will find their equilibrium and you'll feel like a lover, not just a mother.

dealing with negative emotions

It's paramount that you face up to any trauma associated with the pregnancy or birth. Most psychotherapists can trace a link between a disappointing post-baby sex life and a bad birth. At some level you may be scared of sex in case you fall pregnant again and have to repeat the birth; or you may harbour resentment that sex can lead to so much more upheaval for you than for your partner. Either way, unresolved fear or resentment about sex can both contribute to, and be symptomatic of, postnatal depression and should be explored by a health professional.

coping with your hormones

After exhaustion and sharing out your body, there are also hormonal factors to consider. Mother Nature wants to ensure you focus on raising the baby you've got before making any more. This means there's a definite re-entry date for your libido.

physical problems

And even if you've got past all this, you may still fear irrevocable change from the stretching from the birth. But an unsatisfactory sex life really shouldn't come down to altered sensation. In the first month, yes, there is stretching and bruising, which makes it unadvisable to have full penetrative sex, but from week six onwards, your pelvic floor exercises should begin to restore muscle tone and by the end of three months, the vaginal muscles should be every bit as tight and responsive as they were before the birth.

Occasionally, an episiotomy or tear scar can cause discomfort during penetration. This is known as dyspareunea (see page 283) but it can be easily remedied. A specially trained cranio-sacral expert can perform a fascial unwinding technique. They will be able to unwind the fascial restrictions and help restore comfort and sexual function. I also advocate gentle self-stretching of the lower vaginal muscles with Ayurvedic oils or olive oil with a drop of rose otto. Of course if the scarring is very thick and irregular, you may have to resort to surgery for plastic revision of the vaginal scar, but your doctor will advise you on this. Immediately after the surgical repair heals, it will be necessary to see a cranio-sacral practitioner who is also a doctor or midwife to unwind the new, neater surgical scar and restore full function and, hopefully, your sex life.

body image

With their swelling breasts, luxuriant hair and glowing skin, many women claim to feel beautiful and at their most womanly when they are pregnant. Looking in the mirror and examining the latest changes to their baby bump is a daily adventure. Interestingly – and something which fills me with great joy – many mothers report their pregnancy as one of the first moments in their adult lives when they look at their bodies uncritically, seeing not cellulite, wobbly bits or thread veins, but the beauty and awesome power of what their body can achieve.

I have so many letters from mothers who found pregnancy freed them from the tyranny of body fascism and diets. With a magnificent baby bump to nourish and cultivate, they finally did not have to 'compete' with the unrealistic images of femininity bombarded at them from all quarters.

your body after the birth

But what happens after the birth when you're left with more of a jelly belly than a taut tum? Coping with an altered body image is a tough call for most new mothers because their body *is* initially going to look, and feel, different to before. You may now have a scar or stretchmarks, most probably poor muscle tone and some excess weight, and your ribs and hips may have been pushed out an inch or two.

Even those mothers who are back into their jeans within the week will report problem areas and changes. Pregnancy isn't like a shadow that just slips over and off you without trace. It leaves its mark one way or another. But I fiercely believe that we should be proud of these signs of motherhood. Did you know that in some parts of Africa, a man will choose his wife only if she has already proved her fertility by having his baby?

Motherhood is a blessing and its permanent scars should be worn as badges of honour. Everything else can be restored. Your muscles – which repair and renew every day – will become every bit as taut as you exercise them to be. Excess fat will be shed initially by breastfeeding, and, if necessary, finished off by a short, conservative diet (think: nine months on – nine months off). And the Pilates programme included in this book will tone up your muscles. In fact, by the time your baby is six months old, there will be little left that reveals the momentous journey your body has travelled.

Case History: Kasia

I was overwhelmed when I found out I was pregnant! Even though I had come off the pill and wanted to get pregnant, I didn't quite expect it to happen straightaway! I guess my shock was more or less related to the fact that my husband and I had just bought a house that needed a lot of work. When I told Gowri – a close friend of mine – that I was pregnant, we both burst into tears as we realized I was beginning a new era in my life.

I work as one of Gowri's therapists, and the first thing she said was that she didn't want me to work as a therapist as I needed to preserve all my vital energy just for my baby and myself. This sounded like a prison sentence as I love my work, and in spite of the advice I personally give pregnant mothers, I was determined to work as long as I could into my pregnancy. Gowri sat me down on several occasions and explained that we had to protect my baby's stress levels within my womb and that I had to think about my birth process and start preparing for the birth.

All these facts played on my subconscious mind. Even though I had good intentions of following the gentle birth method, I noted that I wanted to eat much more than I usually do, and I seemed to gravitate towards carbohydrates. I put this down to the fact that I was tired and stressed about the work on my house. I was receiving pregnancy treatments and listening daily to the self-hypnosis and visualization tapes for birth preparation.

But I did the same thing a lot of pregnant mothers do, and consoled myself by indulging in carbohydrates. By the time I was twenty weeks pregnant I had already put on two stones in weight and started to slow down. I stopped working hands-on from my twenty-sixth week, and from twenty-eight weeks onwards I thought I was eating healthily. However, despite receiving relaxing treatments, I still felt stressed and often ate takeaways or sugary things. Nevertheless, I kept a very positive mental attitude to the birth and prepared as best as I could. Luckily, all went well and I gave birth to my baby girl so well that I was back home from hospital the very same day. I had a gorgeous baby, an intact perineum and I was so exhilarated that I felt like a queen!

My regret that I had put on too much weight was surpassed by the fact that my birth gave me something to be proud about – I focused on my beautiful baby and slowly began to feel great about my body. All my life I had worked really hard to maintain my size ten figure, but four months after giving birth, I am still a size sixteen. Funnily, I feel a lot better about my body image than I would have thought. My birth was so amazing that everything else seems unimportant. I'm glad to admit that perhaps I am naturally supposed to be a size fourteen. And, strange though it may sound, I feel as if I'm a nicer person within my new postnatal body. My husband and I have bonded deeply with each other and our new baby, and I feel so loved that I can truly say I love my body as it is, and I will be toning it up gently as I go along.

breastfeeding

Breastfeeding merits particular mention here because there tends to be a trouble spot at between three and six months. Remember, successful breastfeeding relies as much upon mental confidence as physical ability, and you'll be thrown a curve ball at this point which may take you off guard. At the three- to four-month mark, your baby's weight gain slows down, but coincides with a growth spurt which makes her want to feed more. The result is usually confusion for the mother who mistakes her baby's weight plateau and apparent hunger for an inadequate milk supply. That's rarely the case – initially.

On top of all this, any time between four and six months your baby will start to show signs of wanting solids.

starting solids

Once your baby starts solids, you will begin to drop feeds, and this is where the problems really dig in. Up until now, your body will have regulated your milk supply quite easily because your baby will have cultivated a consistent demand. However, once you start to drop feeds, the message is sent to the brain to begin to drop that supply. If you are intending to breastfeed beyond weaning (past six months*) you will find that for a short period during this transition phase, you will actually have to become more proactive about it.

* The World Health Organization recommends breastfeeding alongside other foods up to two years of age.

maintaining your milk supply

One way to ensure your milk supply continues is to watch your diet – it becomes as important now as in the first month. Your calorie intake becomes more important. Your brain needs to keep receiving messages to continue producing milk, and a plentiful energy supply will ensure this, as will good rest periods. When you do introduce solids, ensure you offer the breastfeed first. Remember to indulge in some regular reflexology (see page 188) and if you feel you need an extra boost, try some homeopathic Lactors (see Resources). These precautions will all help maintain your milk supply.

dropping milk feeds

Ultimately, weaning will introduce only three main meals, so you can easily retain two or three breastfeeds too (first thing in the morning, post-lunch nap, bedtime). And you can drop feeds very slowly – over a period of months if you like.

When you do choose to drop a feed, you can actually be a bit clever about it. Be strategic in which one you drop first to help 'bump up' the following feed. This will ensure that even though you are feeding less, your supply remains high.

With prolonged breastfeeding you'll find you become expert as to when you have your best quality milk and when you have most milk. You'll probably find that the baby drinks deeply at some feeds and merely snacks at others. Generally speaking, the quality of milk is best first thing in the morning, after a rejuvenating night's sleep, and the quality and quantity generally diminishes throughout the course of the day. So you may want to follow this schedule for dropping feeds (these are average timings based on a 7am–7pm day; adjust to your own schedule as necessary):

drop first:

 i) 11am/12pm feed – when you start weaning, most health visitors recommend this becomes the first solid meal (lunch). The 11am/12pm milk will help boost the 3pm milk.

 ii) 3pm feed – this pushes the 3pm milk to boost the 7pm feed, which tends to have the most compromised milk as you're tired at the end of the day.

 iii) 7pm – many babies find it easier and quicker to feed from the bottle at this age (six months plus).

 iv) 7am feed – this should be the last feed to drop as it has the best-quality milk and you usually have lashings of it after your long night's sleep.

Mothers often like to continue breastfeeding at least in the morning or evening for many months to come. This will provide valuable nutrients and immunological benefits, and is also a time for the mother and baby to snuggle and reconnect.

mother's care

- **Massage.** After six months, you'll find it difficult to remember life without a baby, and your days and nights will feel natural again, but in this last stage, protect your confidence and morale with a massage treatment. Daily massage is ideal, but otherwise aim for three to four times a week. A lovely mix of essential oils is four drops each of rose otto, lavender and lime or lemon, together with two drops of anise. Mix in 30ml of base oil, such as sunflower seed or virgin olive oil.
- **Reflexology.** Ask your partner to perform some firm strokes along the tendons of the upper aspect of your feet (this relates to the breast lymphatic areas). This will help improve lactation.

- **Sleep.** Make a point of getting lots of early nights, even though your baby should begin to sleep through and you may want to stay up later. Aim for at least eight hours a night until you feel fully recovered.

- **Sex.** If your libido has not made a full comeback, I recommend the Ayurvedic herb Ashwagandha, one capsule twice a day (see Resources). This can be very useful during different phases of your life but especially in the period between breastfeeding and weaning. If you feel dry or sore during sex, you may want to use a lubricating agent such as KY Jelly. This will replace the natural vaginal moisture which can diminish during the postnatal year until hormone levels return to normal.

- **Talk to your partner.** If you have yet to resume sexual relations with your partner, keep communication channels open. Discuss it openly. After having launched into parenthood, there may well need to be a more conscious effort to be intimate. Even just these discussions can make your partner feel you are being 'returned' from the baby back to him.

- **Pelvic floor.** You should have full muscle tone in your pelvic floor by now. If you still feel slightly stretched or weak, or are suffering from stress incontinence, then you need extra help. Please see your GP, health visitor or a postnatal physiotherapist who can prescribe some specialist exercises you can practise at home – some may involve intra-vaginal equipment; others may be based on weights.

- **Exercise.** Your general exercise routine can become a little more challenging now. Please continue to avoid high-impact sports if you are breastfeeding, but you will benefit from using light weights for resistance training. These will improve your strength and muscle tone, helping you to firm up and bring back your figure. Do attend more yoga and Pilates classes every month as this will maintain your flexibility and build lean tissue (see Pilates exercise routine, page 191). Daily brisk walks with the pram, cycling, rowing or swims for a minimum of twenty minutes will burn off fat.

- **Listen to my postnatal exercise visualization tape.** It will give you confidence and the belief that you will get your figure back again (see Resources).
- **Take stock and scrutinize your appearance.** It'll be a few weeks before you start noticing changes to your figure, but grooming has an immediate impact. Get your hair cut or highlighted; treat yourself to a manicure and a pedicure. It will give you some valuable – and necessary – time away from the baby and you'll get an instant ego boost.
- **Put away your maternity clothes.** If they're all that fits you, buy a few cheap pieces to carry you over until you drop a size. You'll feel much better to pack away those stretchy panels and elasticated waists.
- **Weight.** Strike a middle ground with your attitude to your weight. You may have lost some of the baby fat by now! Studies have shown that the majority of cases of obesity in women stem from pregnancy, and that if the weight is not lost by six months, it won't ever be. It's good to bear this in mind in case you're reaching for the doughnuts, but for as long as you are breastfeeding, your milk supply must come first. If you want to lose weight, you must do it very, very gently and slowly. The best thing you can do is to step up your daily exercise and go for more walks or swims. And face up to your diet – if you've started snacking on sweets and sugary foods for instant energy, then cut them out without delay. Instead eat five small meals a day, including a good protein balance. But please remember the epithet: nine months on, nine months off. Many mothers find their bodies have naturally shrunk down to something like normality by the nine-month mark. Your baby will love you just as you are. My advice is to go back to my prenatal 'no wheat, no sugar' policy. I can vouch that any excess pounds you may have will drop off rapidly!

pilates routine from three to six months

You should have been doing the Pilates programme for the past six weeks now. The following Pilates moves are to be included into that initial routine as you progress. Build up slowly, listen to your body, and breathe. You will feel different each day, some days you will have more energy than others, so let your body flow in to each position without pushing or pulling.

1: REST POSITION

Aim: This position can be used at any time during the programme. It is a great way to relax and allow the spine to stretch.

Kneel back on your haunches, with your toes extended.

Keeping your buttocks on the heels as much as possible, slowly breathe out and curl the spine forward while sliding your fingers on the floor ahead of you (Fig. 1).

Stretch all the way forward through your fingertips, while pressing your shoulder blades to your hips, forehead rested on the floor. Breathe in without moving. Relax in this position.

Be aware: If there is any discomfort in the knees, place a cushion behind them. This will keep the buttocks off the heels, and allow for a more comfortable stretch.

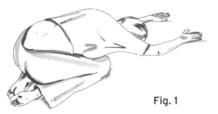

Fig. 1

2: CAT STRETCH

Aim: Flexion mobility for the spine.

Kneel on all fours, hands and knees shoulder-width apart. The centre of each knee should be in line with the second toe; the middle finger should align with the centre of the wrist. Lengthen up through the arms, pulling your shoulders away from your ears, keeping them relaxed, not hunched. Keep your hips square and lower spine lengthened, but flat (Fig. 2).

Breathe out as you slowly draw the head to the groin while pressing the spine to the ceiling. Listen to your body and do not tense your shoulders.

Breathe in, lengthening through the spine as you release the ribs away from the hips until the spine is horizontal to the floor.

Repeat ten times.

Be aware: If there is too much mobility in the upper back, concentrate more on drawing the hips to the ribs.

Go back into rest position, and then slowly come into a seated position, rolling through the spine as you sit up.

Fig. 2

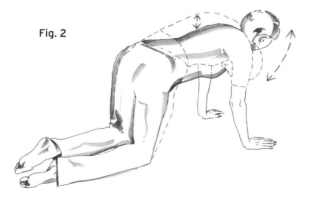

gentle first year

3: THE SAW

Aim: This movement works on the mobility and stretch of your upper back.

Sit on the front of your sit bones, legs hip-width apart, the centre of each knee in line with the second toe, feet flexed.

Lift the ribs away from the hips. Stretching the crown of your head to the ceiling and keeping the shoulders relaxed, take your arms out to the side (Fig. 3).

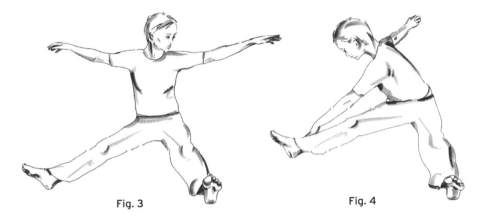

Fig. 3   Fig. 4

Inhale as you lengthen through the spine, then breathe out and turn your body to the side. Keep your arms in line with your shoulders as you turn, and keep your hips facing the front.

Continue to breathe out as you take the outside of your hand to the outside of your knee and slowly slide the hand down the outside of your leg (Fig. 4). Breathe in as you come back to the centre and repeat in the opposite direction on the other side. Repeat ten times.

Be aware: Listen to your breath and body. Relax into the stretch. Do not struggle to touch your toes – build up to it slowly. If you feel an ache in your lower back, bend your knees slightly. You can also place a small towel under your sitting bones to raise your body at an angle.

4A: ROLL-UP ALTERNATIVES

Aim: This variation on the following exercise allows you to start at a lower level. As your strength builds and the flexibility in your back improves, you will be able to take the movement to the full roll-up. Remember to keep your feet on the ground.

Start from a seated position, knees bent, feet shoulder-width apart. Lift the ribs up and away from your hips, arms stretched out in front of you, shoulders relaxed (Fig. 5).

Breathe in as you lengthen through the spine. As you breathe out, scoop your tailbone away from you as you roll down, drawing your lower abs towards your spine (Fig. 6). Breathe in as you return, lengthening through the spine, keeping your movement flowing. Roll down slowly in stages; as your strength builds, you can go down further.

Repeat ten times.

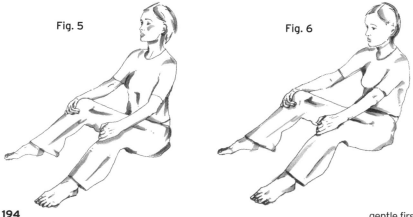

Fig. 5

Fig. 6

Aim: Progression from last move.

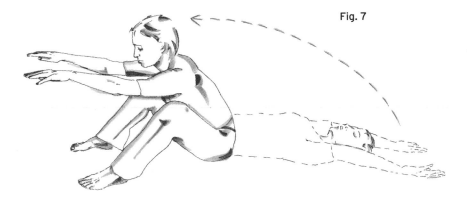

Fig. 7

Lie on the floor with your legs bent. Inhale, extending your arms over your head. As you exhale, slowly bring your arms back over your head, lifting with the chest and slowly peeling your spine off the mat. Stretch out over your legs as you breathe in (Fig. 7). Keep your movements and breathing continuous.

Repeat ten times.

5: SIDE LEG LIFTS

Aim: To strengthen the side muscles of the waist, the oblique abdominal muscles and the outside of the thigh.

Lie on your left side with your head resting on your left arm, elbow in line with the body. Place your right hand lightly on the floor in front of your naval. Keep the legs parallel, slightly in front of the body with toes pointed. There should be a small gap between the left side of the waist and the floor. Tuck the pelvis (posteriorly) to assist in maintaining a flatter back.

Engage centre as you breathe out, lift both legs as high as you can without leaning the hips backwards (Fig. 8).

Breathe in as you lower the legs.

Repeat ten times, then change sides.

Be aware: If there is an arch in the back, flatten this by connecting the lower abdominal muscles more with the posterior tuck. If there is still a fair-sized arch, keep both legs further forward of the straight line of the body, so the back is relaxed.

Fig. 8

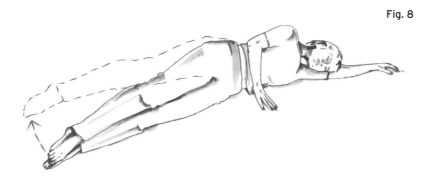

Aim: To tighten the pelvic floor.

You may sit, stand or adopt the relaxation position (see Chapter 2) for this exercise.

Tighten and draw up the pelvic floor, like a flower closing at the end of the day. Then gradually release the muscles, letting them open like a flower in the morning sun.

Be aware: Do not squeeze your buttocks. Think of gently drawing up the internal muscles.

six months to one year

baby
weaning

Weaning strikes fear into the heart of every new mother. Even the gourmet cook whose soufflés never collapse worries about feeding her baby apple purée. Partly this is because breastfeeding will have become so effortless that you will have nourished and nurtured your baby without really thinking about it. But as with most aspects of parenting, weaning really is quite easy when you know how – honest!

The World Health Organization (WHO) recommends that an infant should be exclusively breastfed until six months of age, when weaning should begin. In many countries, however, mothers start introducing other foods to the baby from four months onwards. So how can you tell if your baby really is ready to start weaning?

when to start

Your baby will let you know, in no uncertain terms, when he's ready for solids. Clear signs that your baby is ready for more substance are:

- Uncharacteristic early-morning wakings
- Fussing at the bottle

- Dribbling
- Crying at the end of feeds
- Watching others eat
- Low-grade irritability

And these behavioural symptoms usually occur only after the following developmental stages:

- The ability to sit up
- A fading of the tongue reflex (so your baby doesn't just push solids out of his mouth with his tongue)
- Readiness to chew
- Ability to pick up food and put it in his mouth

But regardless of what your baby is telling you, there is much debate over when is exactly the right time to introduce solids – start too early and you risk overloading an immature digestive system, increasing the risk of allergies; start too late and your baby may be a fussier eater. WHO and Department of Health guidelines are that babies should be weaned at about six months, but if you do begin to wean before six months, make sure the following indicators apply:

- Your baby has doubled his birth weight
- He weighs over 16lb
- He is older than 20 weeks

If in any doubt about weaning do talk to your health visitor.

---
weaning equipment

- At least seven soft cloth bibs
- At least seven rubber weaning spoons. These are smaller than teaspoons and soft on toothless gums – most babies hate the feel of metal spoons until they have teeth.
- Three or four small weaning pots with lids. These will allow you to take feeds with you when you go out, and are extra-small to help keep the first tiny portions warm.
- Steam sterilizer. For the first two months, sterilize all the feeding equipment, including spoons. After then, you will be fine so long as the utensils are put through the dishwasher. You will need to continue sterilizing bottles until the baby is one year.

---

first foods

There are a couple of things to bear in mind before you begin:

1 Only introduce one solid meal at a time.
2 Continue to offer the breastfeed before the solid tasters, so that the baby's milk intake remains stable.

Ideally, you want to introduce new meals at opposite ends of the day, so that the baby is sufficiently nourished whilst learning to process solid food in his mouth. Remember, the first weeks are about tasting, not filling.

Remember, the first weeks are about tasting, not filling.

BABY RICE

Begin by mixing a small teaspoon of baby rice (available from all supermarkets and good pharmacies) with either expressed breast milk or formula. The consistency should be gloopy and binding enough to stay on the weaning spoon. It should also be warm. Baby rice is so bland that, when cold, it is very unappealing. Your baby may well take only two to four mouthfuls on the first few attempts. You're getting him used to trying new flavours, and also teaching him how to open his mouth for the spoon and move the food with his tongue from the front to the back of his mouth (a very different technique from breast- and bottle-feeding). Initially, his instinct will be to thrust the food straight back out with his tongue, but persevere (and buy lots of bibs!) and just bear in mind that early weaning is very much a case of one step forward, two steps back.

After two or three days, introduce a mild fruit purée such as pear or apple, and mix it in with the baby rice. You'll probably find the baby loves this new, sweet, bolder flavour, and having begun to get the hang of spoon-feeding, will accept it more readily.

After then, you're off. Allow three days for the baby to accept a new taste, and alternate offering fruit with vegetable purées to discourage him from developing only a sweet tooth – so pear, followed by carrot, followed by apple, followed by courgette and so on.

I recommend the following foods in the first two months of weaning.

FRUIT

- Cooked or puréed pear, apple, peach, plum, kiwi fruit. All of these fruits can be given as whole meals in themselves, or mixed with baby rice.
- Quinoa (tiny fruits that looks like a grain). Boiled and mashed, it makes great baby food. It has the added advantage of being high in protein. You can use it as a base for mixing with mashed and cooked vegetables.

VEGETABLES

- Carrots
- Green beans
- Sweet potato
- Swede
- Parsnip
- Courgette
- Butternut squash

FRUIT AND VEGETABLES TO AVOID

- **Strawberries** (allergenic)
- **Bananas.** Some of the varieties available in supermarkets cause constipation as they have been artificially ripened using chemicals. In India, ripe bananas are actually given to help the bowel move along. Babies love bananas but I advise only ripe, organic bananas mashed with another fruit (such as kiwi fruit) to prevent constipation.
- **Tomatoes** belong to the nightshade family, as do potatoes, and are not totally desirable as they may affect the immune system.
- **Shellfish** (high risk of food poisoning)
- **Soft cheeses** may contain mould and bacteria, especially if they are unpasteurized.

- **Oranges** (too acidic)

For the first two months of weaning, any food with skins – grapes, peaches, apples, plums, sweetcorn – should be peeled or put through a food processor as your baby will not yet have enough teeth to mash the skins.

---

weaning tip

If your baby doesn't like a particular taste, slightly increase the amount of baby rice mixed in so that it is milder and less offensive.

STORING AND FREEZING PURÉES

When you have cooked and blended the purées, decant them into ice cube trays in the freezer, before storing them in separate freezer bags. When required, defrost the quantity required overnight, ready for the next day. Initially, your baby will only take one cube of purée, but will build up to three to four by the time you introduce proteins in two months.

MICROWAVING

Please refrain from microwaving your baby's food as it has been shown that microwaving can change the molecular structure of food. There is evidence that the body can't really distinguish between different types of food when they are microwaved. This causes confusion: the digestive glands do not know which kind of enzymes to secrete, leading to overactivity and exhaustion. It is well known to the medical community that cellular exhaustion can lead to chronic health problems.

THIRST

Thirst is a new impulse to deal with when weaning. Your baby's hydration will have been satisfied with every milk feed. Solids will make your baby more thirsty, so offer sips of water throughout the day.

Tap water should have been boiled and allowed to cool first and, if possible, filtered with a simple filter jug (like a Brita filter – available from many supermarkets). Prepare a covered jug each morning to use throughout the day. Serve at room temperature because ice-cold water shocks the baby's pancreas and interferes with the normal secretion of digestive enzymes. Avoid mineral waters as some of them have high levels of sodium and added chlorine that can be harmful to babies' bodies.

timing

Most health visitors advise introducing the first solid meal at the 11am/12pm feed, as this will give you the rest of the day to see if the baby reacts favourably to a new food, without the risk of disturbing his sleep. Equally, most babies are ravenous at breakfast time and just want calories quickly. They are less likely to wait to savour new flavours at that time – and anyway, who wants courgette for breakfast?

When you start to introduce 'solids' you will find that your baby automatically starts to take less breast milk and that your supply reduces over time.

After five to seven days of gentle weaning, you can introduce a second solid meal, this time for supper (around 5pm). If your baby is happy with a meal – such as baby rice with puréed apple – bump this back to suppertime (5pm) and introduce a new vegetable purée for lunch. Organize the roster so that the baby is eating both sweet and savoury foods over the course of the day.

When your baby is more fully weaned, make a conscious effort to offer more savoury than sweet foods – more vegetables than fruits – and never give sweets, chocolates, ice creams, fizzy drinks or fruit juices. The only time I recommend fruit juice is if the baby is ill and vomiting – very dilute juice will keep the baby hydrated, and the extra calories can prove useful – but otherwise the foods and drinks listed above have zero nutritional benefits for your baby and should be strictly avoided. (Note: You may well find that the baby wants to be breastfed more when he is ill and recovering. This is good for the baby, providing the extra calories he needs and antibodies from you.)

allergies

Watch for and note down any allergic reactions to new foods such as:

- Red patches
- Blotchiness
- Hives
- Itching
- Sneezing
- Wheezing

More extreme reactions such as breathlessness or swelling of the tongue require *immediate* medical help, as your child may be having an anaphylactic reaction. This is very serious and you need to take your baby to hospital straight away. When there is a serious anaphylactic reaction, the doctors will have to inject the baby with steroids and adrenaline to prevent life-threatening bronchospasm.

If your baby does appear to be allergic to some foods or food groups, make an appointment with your health visitor and ensure the allergies are recorded in your child's GP records and red book. Sometimes, allergies can be lessened by a desensitizing programme of regular exposure to minuscule amounts of the offending substances, usually as skin patches. These programmes are carried out by specialists, and your GP will refer you.

nuts

Nuts - especially peanuts, pistachios and cashews - should be avoided until your child is five years old. These are common allergens and avoiding them in childhood may reduce the likelihood of allergies later on in life.

PROTEINS

Protein foods have a much stronger taste than anything your baby has experienced before. Introduce protein gently by mixing some organic chicken stock with baby rice for a couple of days. After that, move on to a soft – preferably organic – chicken soup.

Once you have introduced protein, you can begin to cook more 'composite' meals such as spaghetti bolognese and roast chicken, which combine all the tastes you've experimented with in the first two months. This makes it easier for you, as you can cook meals for the rest of the family and just whizz up the baby's portion in the blender.

TEXTURE

Gradually introduce more texture to your baby's foods as soon as you think he will be able to handle it. The sooner you train his palate, the more fun eating will become. Start first with fruit – mash it and serve it raw after two months – then once he's comfortably 'gumming' the food (mashing it between the gums) move on to other food groups.

---

ingredients to avoid

Salt. Remember never to add any seasoning - especially salt - to any food the baby will be sharing. For the foreseeable future, get into the habit of seasoning at the table, not the stove.

Sugar. Don't add sugar to food.

Honey. Honey has been implicated as being infected with bacteria that release toxins. Recently a whole batch of honey from China was taken off supermarket shelves in the UK. There is also a strong link with infant botulism if honey is given before the baby is one year old.

---

meal ideas

Fish Pie

Make fish pie with cod, halibut or fresh haddock, and some mashed peas or sweetcorn. Top the pie with a thin layer of mashed potatoes, sprinkle with a fine layer of Cheddar cheese, and bake.

Spaghetti Bolognese

Cook 100g of finely ground steak mince for about fifteen minutes with a small, finely chopped onion in a little vegetable soup (used as an oil substitute). Then drop a handful of vermicelli, preferably wheat-free, or 'angel hair' (wonderfully fine) pasta into a small saucepan of boiling water and allow to simmer for about seven minutes or till cooked. Drain the water and gently stir in the cooked meat.

Quinoa and Vegetables

Quinoa is a South American superfood, a fruit that looks like a grain. Boil for twenty minutes, drain and then mix with cooked and mashed vegetables such as butternut squash, peas or beetroot. Serve seasoned with a dash of olive oil and, if you wish, a squeeze of lemon.

Mung Dhal with Rice

Take half a teacup of mung dhal and soak in water for twenty-four hours. Then drain the water, add one-and-a-half cups of fresh water and allow to boil for half an hour till almost a paste. This is highly nutritious and very easy to digest. Serve on its own or mixed half-and-half with overcooked soft rice. Add a teaspoon of ghee (clarified butter). A portion for a six-month-old will be about four tablespoons.

Avocado and Egg

Boil the egg for four minutes and mash it up with half a ripe avocado. Add a drop of lemon juice and serve!

Rice and Dhal with Sun-ripened Organic Bananas or Mangoes

Mash one small banana or a few slices of very ripe mango with a small cupful of overcooked rice. Add two tablespoons of dhal, boiled and cooked with turmeric till very soft. Mix everything together and serve. This was an all-time favourite in my home when we were growing up.

Recipe for Chicken Stew

1 small onion, finely chopped
2 teaspoons of sunflower oil
2 cloves
2 peppercorns
2.5cm (1-inch) stick of cinnamon
Handful of organic chicken, finely diced
1 small carrot, grated
285ml (½ pint) of boiling water
Dash of turmeric
2 teaspoons of cornflour dissolved in 2 tablespoons of water

1 Sauté the onion in the sunflower oil. Then add the cloves, peppercorns and cinnamon. Sauté for about three to five minutes till you get an aromatic smell.
2 Add the chicken and sauté for another three minutes.
3 Then add the carrot, boiling water and turmeric. Bring all of this to a boil and allow to simmer for 30 minutes.
4 Finally add the dissolved cornflour and bring to the boil, stirring all the while till you see the mixture thicken. Cool and serve warm.

Grilled or Baked Vegetables

These are simple to make. Cut strips of vegetables like parsnips, carrots, red peppers, thinly sliced potato, butternut squash, runner beans, a few slices of aubergine. Lay them on a baking tray and drizzle all over with olive oil. Bake in a preheated oven for about twenty to thirty minutes till all the vegetables look cooked. This makes great finger food and is delicious. Sprinkle with feta cheese for three minutes before removing from the oven.

Egg Boats

Hard-boil four eggs and cut them into quarters. Scoop out the firm yolks and mix with a tablespoon of butter and a teaspoon of grated cheese while still warm. This will make a nice paste-like mixture. Spoon this mixture into a piping bag or wide icing nozzle and pipe into the hollow part of the egg quarters. Create the sails to your boats by slicing carrots into very small, flat, triangular pieces, and decorate the egg boats with these sails. Arrange your egg boats on a decorative plate like a fleet and watch them disappear!

Almost every mother has her own version of interesting food. Be creative. Enjoy!

separation anxiety

Up until now, your baby has revelled in the security of life as a two-headed, four-armed and twenty-toed creature, but his growing physical independence will have gradually made him aware that actually only ten of those fingers are his; the rest are yours – and you can take them away with you whenever you want. It's an overwhelming realization for your baby, but also monumental. The *raison d'être* of parenting lies in nurturing your child to confident, contented, compassionate independence, and separation anxiety is the very necessary – albeit painful – mental leap that allows this to happen.

The age of onset varies widely but it usually surfaces any time from six months, peaking at eighteen months and ebbing away by three years. There are two key steps to resolving separation anxiety:

1 **Coming to grips with object permanence – understanding that an object (i.e. you) continues to exist even when it is not in view.**
2 **Experience – realizing that even though you may go away, you always return to him.**

Until separation anxiety kicks in, babies inhabit an 'out of sight, out of mind' world. While they are undoubtedly delighted to see you, they will not necessarily have pined or even much noticed that you weren't there previously, so long as their needs were met. It may hurt your feelings to realize this initially, but it's only with hindsight that you'll see that such ignorance was bliss.

how to handle separation anxiety

Unfortunately, separation anxiety is like teething – it comes and goes in episodes over many months, and usually gets worse before it gets better – but the learning curve can be accelerated if you handle it correctly and sensitively. Although it's wearing being greeted with screams every time you turn your back, it's important to understand that this marks the beginning of the end of that intense – even claustrophobic – period when you are inextricably entwined with your baby's sense of self. There are usually a lot of tears before he comes to realize (every mother's secret) that actually *he* is intrinsic to *your* sense of self!

Trust and confidence are the key words. When you do have to leave him for short periods, make sure you have communicated where you are going, who will be looking after him, and that you will be coming back. Affectionate but brief goodbyes are best, and hold your nerve even if he's sobbing. Remember, object permanence isn't fully established yet, and it's a rare mummy whose memory can persist after ten minutes, or compete against a bright, bouncy Teletubby! On your return, make a fuss and give a really big greeting: hold your arms wide, cover him in big cuddles and kisses, and shower him with praise for doing so well. Greet him like this every time you go away and he'll remember – and anticipate – your loving returns.

baby care

- From six months, introduce your baby to baby rice mixed with milk before moving on to soft fruits and mashed vegetables such as carrots, peas, courgettes, pears, peaches and plums.
- Introduce a drink of water with solid meals, and for your baby to sip from throughout the day.

- By seven months, your baby will have mastered sitting independently. Once he is sitting confidently, place toys slightly in front of him and to his side to encourage him onto his hands and knees, the first step to crawling.
- During this adventurous period, your baby may well roll over in his cot at night (from back to tummy) but not yet be able to roll back again. This will probably mean a spell of disturbed evenings for you as you have to go and 'rescue' him. Train him by putting him on his tummy a lot during playtimes. The stronger his upper chest and shoulders, the more ably he will roll onto his back again.
- Some of the positions your baby gets into will make your eyes water – sitting with his knees bent inwards (ankles at his hips), or pushing his bottom up so that he is looking between his straight legs. In yoga, these are known as the Cow and Downward Dog positions, but to your baby it's just movement. His joints and muscles are still naturally elastic and flexible, so encourage him by joining in (if you can). He'll love it if you hang upside down and stare back at him through your legs. Baby yoga!
- By eight months, introduce finger foods such as soft carrot or baby sweet corn, cucumber sticks, and baby biscuits.
- Switch to a beaker for your baby's water drink.
- At eight months, you may find your baby is taking longer to settle at his afternoon nap. Keep your 'picking-up time' the same, but put him down three minutes later every other day, so that the nap is foreshortened, and eventually dropped when it is less than ten minutes long.
- Begin to mash raw fruit and leave the skins on (if your baby has enough teeth).
- Crawling is to be highly encouraged – studies have shown that children who do not crawl are more likely to suffer from dyspraxia and dyslexia. Babies can crawl any time from six months, but on average, most master it at ten months. Keep putting him on his hands and knees, and place a favourite toy just out of reach. You could also practise wheelbarrows together (holding his feet whilst he bears his weight on his arms). He'll probably only take a step or two, but there

is a noted parallel between weak upper body strength and dyspraxia, so it's worth trying to build up his strength naturally and encourage crawling to occur.

- When your child is fully crawling, create little obstacle courses for him to navigate – a pile of cushions becomes a magnificent mountain to climb over; or stack up two pillars of cushions, with a larger one across the top (Stonehenge-style) and get him to crawl through it, like a tunnel. Beware though: this dexterity will enable him to climb up the stairs so ensure you have baby-proofed the house with stair gates and cupboard locks, etc.
- Allow your baby to take tours of the house. Having previously been carried through a series of separate rooms, he'll be fascinated to see how they all 'join up'.
- Expandable nylon tunnels can be bought cheaply at toy shops– your baby will love to see your face appear at the other end – but you could also just knock through the ends of a big box. Double the fun by painting it first and sticking on glitter and tissues with him.
- Finger painting will prove highly entertaining at this stage, as he begins to use his hands as instruments.
- Cock your head to one side and wait for your baby to copy you. They love to see the world a different way up.
- Your baby is easily grasping and hitting toys now. The next step is to refine his pincer movement (thumb and index finger) so give him smaller objects – such as sweetcorn at the dinner table – to pick up. Keep a close eye, however, to prevent choking risks.
- Although he is easily reaching toys, he can't yet let go; so give him toys that are rewarding to hold on to, such as maracas or a rainmaker.
- Banging will also be a favourite pastime, so give him a drum, xylophone, or a wooden spoon and saucepan and let him make mad, crazy music. He'll enjoy a hammer and ball set too.
- Sit him in front of a jack-in-the-box and watch him begin to anticipate the 'boo' (check it's a gentle jack-in-the-box – some are a little too enthusiastic and can frighten babies).

- He may be teething with the upper and lower outer central teeth. Give him cold soothers to bite down on, and apply anaesthetic gels to his gums when he seems irritable. If he's an early teether, the molars (or grinding teeth) may begin to come through around the one-year mark.

---

homeopathic teething remedies

- If your baby is cranky, wants to be carried all day and has red swollen gums give camomilla 6C three times a day for five days.
- If teething is accompanied by diarrhoea, with stools that are green and offensive, give calcarea phos 6C three times a day for five days.
- If teething is delayed and accompanied by a sweaty forehead, give calcarea carb 200, three doses at intervals of ten to fifteen minutes, once a week.
- Use the teething pendant (see page 116).

- Introduce your baby to playing in water and baby swim classes at eight to ten months. If you are using a public, cool-water pool, invest in a baby wetsuit first (see Resources), as he will not move much yet, and so will quickly become chilled. Some hospitals and special needs schools hire out their warm-water hydrotherapy pools to specialist baby classes, so make local enquiries.
  - When you get into the water, start by simply supporting your baby around his torso, standing at his side, and swishing him through the water. Give him lots of time to build up confidence – bear in mind the acoustics of swimming pools can amplify noise, and lots of splashing can make little ones panicky. The reflections of the water are also a lot for young eyes to adjust to. If he does seem overwhelmed, cuddle him in close to you and just move slowly through the water together.

- Rhymes he will enjoy now include: 'Humpty Dumpty' (sit him on your knee and whoosh him down when Humpty falls); 'Sing a Song of Sixpence' (pinch his nose when the blackbird takes the maid's nose); 'Incy Wincy Spider' up his legs, arms, tummy...
- Now that he can sit up, encourage more mobility and a sense of fun by raising your arms and wiggling your torso from side to side. He'll love doing the 'wiggly woo' and it's an early form of dancing together.
- Your baby will recognize his name now, as well as other basic words (such as bath, nappy, milk), so sing songs and insert his name in them.
- Sit opposite him and practise waving and clapping. He should be getting really good at it by now, and may even give himself a congratulatory clap if you praise him.
- Shake your hair in front of him. He'll be absolutely thrilled and copy by shaking his head from side to side too.
- He'll enjoy pointing at you and at objects now. This is further progress in communication as he is using his body to show you what he wants. Help him along by responding to what he points out and naming it.
- Your baby may well start cruising and even walking at around one year (although the average age is 14 months). Stand him behind a baby walker and support him under the arms as you help him take some tentative steps. These motor functions will be recorded by the brain and become that little bit easier next time. Encourage him to walk barefoot, as the foot will be more responsive to contact with the floor, and he'll be less likely to slip.
- Stand him in front of you and count '1, 2, 3' then let go. Let him stand unsupported until he begins to wobble forward or his knees bend. Catch him before he falls, as dented confidence will put him off. After a few tries, he'll begin to recognize the counting sequence and anticipate standing on his own.
- Cuddle your baby close and stand next to a mirror together. He'll be nearer to eighteen months before he recognizes the reflection as his, but he'll be bemused to see you – precious mummy – cuddling another baby!

- Swap over his cloth books for board books now. He'll become absorbed in the simple, graphic pictures and be able to turn the pages himself.
- Identify parts of the body to your baby – pat his head and pat yours; squeeze his knees; tap his feet. 'Simon Says' will become lots of fun now, as will dancing the 'Hokey Cokey' together.
- Give him a bead game to play with at the table whilst you prepare his meals. It'll fine-tune his hand-eye coordination as he traces the beads along the wire, and also his fine motor skills (pinching the beads).
- At around twelve months, your baby will understand how to let go of things – cue lots of dropping toys from his highchair. It's frustrating for you, but try to see it as the important milestone it is.
- Put a scented flower like jasmine or honeysuckle under your baby's nose. He won't be able to specifically sniff yet, but just through inhaling as he breathes, he'll take in and notice the scent. Eventually, he'll make the connection between inhaling and smelling, and start consciously to sniff (useful when he gets his next cold).
- Do the same thing with aromatic food too – to encourage him to sniff but also to create a sensual appreciation of food. It'll make him more willing to try new flavours.
- Your baby will understand a lot of what you say by now, but evidence suggests that toddlers – especially boys – find it hard to follow sentences longer than nine words, so keep your communications brief and direct.

mother
returning to work

The biggest upheaval facing you in this period is a possible return to work. Most companies offer a standard six-month maternity leave. In an ideal world, I would prefer my mothers to refrain from work for at least the first year, but I understand that this is often a luxury and not a choice.

For some mothers, returning to work is actually the better option. Now that the learning curve has reached a plateau, the adrenaline has subsided and life has settled down into a routine of play dates and purées, some mothers find themselves itching for just *a bit more*. This is entirely understandable. Much of the stay-at-home mother's day is mundane (which is quite different from boring, quiet or uneventful!) and it can take its toll on some. There are only two crucial issues at stake:

1 **The quality of the time you spend with your baby.**
2 **Making absolutely sure that the person caring for your baby is unimpeachable.**

If you are hiring a nanny, au pair or childminder, or looking at nurseries, every reference must be checked and you must interview exhaustively until you are sure that you have found the right person or place. Satisfy those criteria and you can sleep easy.

On the other hand, if you are able to stay at home with your baby, it's important to stay 'alert' during this calmer period and remain attuned to your baby. (A recent study showed that babies of stay-at-home mothers had only 30 minutes' quality time with their mothers in the day.) It's unrealistic to sit on the floor reading board books and building towers for ten hours of the day, but you should make it a goal to achieve or try something new every day. Try some of these ideas:

- Insert large shapes into a wooden puzzle.
- Stick your fingers in the play dough.
- Paint some pictures for your partner to come home to.
- Go for a splash and swim.
- Dance around the sitting room together.

Your baby will love you for it and you'll realize exactly how lucky you are to share these moments with your baby.

mother's care

- **Biting.** This is common during this stage of breastfeeding, and can be excruciatingly painful. You will learn to anticipate when your baby is about to bite, as he'll pause from feeding and change his position slightly to retract his tongue. Of course, your baby has to learn from your response that it is not acceptable, regardless. The first time he bites, take him off quickly and say that you did not like that. If he repeats the biting, take him off the breast immediately and finish the feed there and then. He will quickly learn that biting leads to an empty stomach. I was told by a wonderful woman, Paradise Newland, who I met in Hawaii that children are unable to hear the word 'no' so she replaced it with 'Zero can do!'

- **Giving up breastfeeding.** Many mothers give up breastfeeding at some point in this period – perhaps due to biting, weaning or returning to work. When you do, you can choose more freely how you eat, drink and exercise. This is the real 'handing over' period for getting your body back. Allow at least a month to six weeks for your hormone levels to return to normal and for your ligaments to tighten up again. In that interim period, concentrate on some core strength moves which will tighten the ligaments and tone the muscles. After six months you can take up more energetic forms of yoga and Pilates, go swimming, skiing or dancing or play tennis. Refrain from running as it does damage your knees eventually.

- **Breast problems.** As you give the baby solids, he will automatically take less breast milk from you, and you will start producing less naturally. However, there is still a risk of engorgement and mastitis, even at this late stage, so be vigilant for lumps, redness or a raised temperature.

- **Alcohol.** You'll find your alcohol tolerance has dropped considerably, so proceed cautiously.

- **Returning to work.** If you are returning to work, place your photo in your baby's cot and let him hear your voice down the phone – he'll be intrigued and the nanny bemused. Give him a big greeting on your return and shower him with affection. Make a point of interacting meaningfully with him before he goes to bed, even if you've only got a few minutes together. Throw off your suit and get in the bath with him, sing a lullaby, read him a bedtime story or do some cupping as he lies in his cot.

- **Aromatherapy baths.** Soak in a rose otto and lavender oil bath or add about six drops of refreshing lime essential oil to your bath at least once a week.

- **Massage.** Try to book a pampering massage treatment at least every six to eight weeks. I do advise all my mothers to have a creative healing female treatment every six months. If you are thinking of conceiving, you should have a creative healing female treatment five days before a period is due. This clears out your fallopian tubes and helps the uterine lining shed all the toxins, even from the deeper layers, and get ready for a healthy implantation.

pre-conceptual care – getting ready for next time
is there a right time to conceive again?

Is that the time already? Many people do begin to think about Number Two (or Three) after their baby's first birthday. Partly, it's because their baby is leaving true babyhood and morphing into a toddler – and from there it's only a wobbly hop, skip and jump to Big School – and some mothers feel wistful to be leaving the baby stage so soon.

There are so very many factors that determine the right time for trying to conceive your next child: the mother's age for starters. If you are over thirty-five and want a medium-to-large family, you may well feel it is preferable to have your babies quickly. After this age your fertility drops and the risk of chromosomal abnormalities rises sharply, so even though it's an exhausting option, many feel it is worth it in the long run.

You may want a small age gap to increase the likelihood of the siblings becoming playmates. There are never any guarantees that your siblings will like each other, but the odds are increased when their abilities and interests overlap. Of course, the downside to this falls on you. Your firstborn, at two, may be walking and possibly talking, but he's still a long way from being a logical, independent being. Chances are he'll still like being carried everywhere, spoon-fed, be in nappies, and prone to throwing fierce tantrums. It's a huge workload and needs consideration.

I'm impressed by the fact that many ancient cultures – and Indian manuscripts written more than three thousand years ago – advise a gap of at least five to seven years between children. Of course in those days women started families earlier in their lives, which meant that a gap of seven years between children could occur. Nowadays, many mothers start their families in their early or mid-thirties, making it difficult to leave such long gaps. However, as the age of reason is supposed to be reached at seven years, and as each child needs so much one-to-one care, I feel there should be a bigger age gap between children if at all possible.

The normal spacing nowadays is about three years. With a three to four-year gap by the time the baby is born, your eldest will be more independent. The older child may well be more conscious of the baby's arrival and react jealously to having you 'taken away' from him. You may also find it harder to come out of your 'comfort zone' of sleeping through the nights. Going back to broken nights, coping with the baby's demands and nappy changes can be a shock.

With a gap of three to four years, going back to broken nights, coping with the baby's demands and nappy changes can be a shock.

For some, the gap between children is determined not by the parents' thoughts on ages, but the time of year they would prefer the baby to be born. I know many mothers who deliberately shy away from having winter babies and choose to give birth in the spring and summer when the nights are shorter and warmer. Somehow, the nights don't feel quite so broken if it gets dark at 10pm and light by 4am.

Completely at the other end of the thought process, some parents choose to have autumn and winter babies expressly for the head start it gives the child at school. With the European school year starting in September and ending in July, those born in September and October have been shown to do better in exams – even at 16 years of age! – than the 'babies' of the year born in July and August.

And absolutely all of these hypotheses about the 'right time' to extend the family are based on the assumption that conception can be determined so precisely. Of course, having children at all is a blessing and not something that should ever be taken for granted. We should remember that every baby is a gift, and ignore the minutiae surrounding dates and ages. At the end of the day, months and years just become statistics!

optimizing your health for conception

When you are ready to start trying for another baby, follow these recommendations to optimize your pre-conceptual health:

- Take 5mg of folic acid a day pre-conceptually and all the way through pregnancy to reduce the risk of congenital abnormalities such as spina bifida, and also to reduce miscarriage risk. I recommend the Biocare or Solgar ranges.
- Eat more dark-green leafy vegetable such as broccoli, green cabbage, Swiss chard and spinach leaves. If possible, juice them.
- Take steam baths in the first half of your cycle, before ovulation, to help sweat out the heavy metals from your system. Infra-red sauna cabins (see Resources) can help you sweat out heavy metals and cholesterol. Avoid steam baths after you think you have ovulated because if you are pregnant, raising the body's temperature in a steam room might induce a miscarriage. For the same reason, avoid saunas or Jacuzzis in the second half of your cycle.
- One of the reasons I mention heavy metals is that many of us have been given amalgam fillings by dentists. There is good evidence to suggest that too many mercury ions or other heavy metals in the circulation can suppress ovulation and cause toxic conditions within the lining of the womb, preventing implantation. In my work at the Essex fertility clinic, I have had many mothers fall pregnant almost immediately after they finished replacing their amalgam fillings. Of course, during the course of dental treatment they were supported by a vitamin and mineral detox.

- See your local reflexologist and ask them to concentrate on detoxifying and clearing your pelvic lymphatics, and stimulating your ovarian reflexes as well as your hypothalamus. As a general rule, avoid reflexology in the last week of your cycle, just in case you are implanting and an energetic treatment might trick your body into believing that you want to shed your uterine lining.
- Consult the Ayurvedic chart (see Chapter 2) to get an idea of your *dosha*:
  - If you are predominantly *vata* you could do a self-massage. Take some olive oil and warm it gently, and then massage your limbs in a downward direction. You can mix four drops of lavender oil in about 30ml of base oil.
  - If you are predominantly *pitta*, avoid steam baths altogether and have milk baths with 2 pints of milk added to a bathful of lukewarm water (about 34 degrees centigrade). Also eat a small ramekin full of homemade rice pudding daily – made with overcooked rice and semi-skimmed goat's milk, with a teaspoon of maple syrup to taste. This cools you down!
  - If you are predominantly *kapha*, avoid sweet foods. Self-massage and light exercise will stimulate your lymphatics and get you birth fit.
- If you had a Caesarean previously and would like a vaginal birth this time, it's important to optimize your skin's health. Cranial osteopaths can unwind the scar to make it thinner and less ropey, making the scar itself healthier and therefore stronger. Alternatively, you can try this at home:

- Make a mixture in a small bottle: add ten drops of essential oil of tea tree and lavender and/or tangerine oil to 30ml virgin olive oil. Take about a teaspoon of this and massage it into your old Caesarean scar area. Lift, roll and very gently knead the tissues beneath your scar with your fingers. As you work on the scar between your fingers, visualize the thick tissues slowly melting away to be replaced with normal-feeling tissues.
- Repeat every day for two to three minutes. You may feel the lightening up of your scar within a month.

- Get plenty of 'good fats', or omega oils, in your diet. Apart from the positive effects on your central nervous system, these will also improve your skin's condition, so make sure you are taking enough. Your ratio of omegas 3, 6, 9 should be 2:1:1. Snack on sunflower or pumpkin seeds, oily fish such as herrings, mackerel and sardines, or take fish oil supplements. Reputable brands include Mother Hemp oil, Dr Udo's oil capsules or the Biocare range.
- Cut down your alcohol and caffeine intake, as both of these cause adrenal exhaustion. This might give rise to problems during your next pregnancy in terms of swellings in your legs and systemic exhaustion, with a tendency to high blood pressure.
- I hope it goes without saying – please refrain from smoking. Chromosomal abnormalities, stillbirths and cot death are significantly higher in babies whose mothers smoked during pregnancy. Your partner should also cut out smoking, reduce his alcohol intake and improve his diet.
- Ask your partner to perform a creative healing pelvic drainage and, if possible, the female treatment five days before a period is due. This will help your tubes to be clear for your next cycle.(See Resources for a creative healing fertility workshop DVD.)
- Take 500mg of vitamin C daily. This will optimize cell division, helping the embryo to implant in the womb, and boost the development of the baby and the placenta.

- Make sleep a priority again. A rested body is more likely to conceive than an exhausted, stressed one.
- Ayurvedic herbs can boost both yours and your partner's libido. Take one capsule of Ashwagandha twice a day. The mother-to-be should take one capsule of Shatavari twice a day, as it is a great hormone balancer.
- Bring down your exercise routine. Cut out contact sports and reduce high-impact activities, such as running, tennis, badminton, skating, horse-riding, scuba diving and skiing. You can carry on cycling, rowing and walking. Even if you are a regular and seasoned yoga devotee, cut out certain forms of strenuous yoga (like Ashtanga or Bickram yoga). And if you do get pregnant, refrain from yoga in the first sixteen weeks till your baby's placenta has safely implanted. I have noticed that in the West, we need to respect the fact that yoga is supposed to be done in a relaxed manner. Improper yoga creates difficulties in the birth process.

Did you do this much work last time, just to get pregnant? Probably not! But then if you've learnt anything over the past year, and the nine months before that, it's probably that when it comes to babies, you can never do too much. Preparation gives you confidence, calm, control – and the opportunity to reframe previous experiences.

Your second pregnancy is going to feel so different to your first. In comparison with last time, you've already got a Degree in Baby (and by following the gentle method, you should have graduated with honours). You already know the journey you are about to embark upon – the joys and the challenges! But you also know the happy ending – the reward of a bouncing bonny baby who makes your heart grow larger every day and fills you with joy! This brief period of growing and raising your family is the best of times, so love your partner, love your babies, love your life – and go forth and multiply!

a note for your next birth

From my extensive understanding of what a woman needs during labour, I advocate choosing a birth supporter who is very well informed about all aspects of pregnancy and childbirth, as well as being trained in several holistic therapies. It is my wish that every midwife should undergo training to be a gentle birth method practitioner. But until that happens, try to find a midwife who will come to your home as soon as possible when you call to inform her that the contractions have started. She should attend you all the way, performing routine midwifery checks on you and the baby. At the appropriate time, if you intend to give birth in hospital, she should then accompany you to the hospital and continue helping the birth process by giving you treatments such as reflexology, Bowen pelvic release moves and creative healing massage. She would also talk you through visualization of your birth process and administer relevant homeopathic remedies to calm and support you. The final delivery would be totally satisfying for all involved.

mother & baby health a-z

In this chapter you will find listed some of the most common postnatal conditions for both mother and baby. Suggestions for treating these conditions are given. Most can be treated with homeopathy, so please read the following guidance before proceeding.

how to take homeopathic remedies

It is best not to eat or drink anything except water for ten minutes before and after taking a remedy, and to let the remedy dissolve under the tongue. In practice, this may be difficult with babies so avoid feeding around the time of giving the remedy. You may find it easier to crush the remedy between two clean teaspoons (use two tablets as some will inevitably be lost or left on the spoon). Add a couple of drops of water to the powder and give this solution to the baby.

For treating acute illness at home, unless otherwise specified, follow these guidelines:

- The potencies advised for home use in this book are 12x and 30c.
- The more urgent the situation, the more often the remedy needs to be repeated.

- You may need to repeat the remedy every five to fifteen minutes at first, if the illness has come on suddenly and there is a lot of pain; less frequently if the symptoms have developed more slowly and are less severe. Stop on improvement. Repeat if the same symptoms return, and repeat as needed to sustain improvement.
- Change the remedy if there has been no improvement after several doses.
- Change the remedy if the symptoms' picture changes.
- Consult a homeopath if the illness does not respond, or if in any doubt.

I appreciate the advice given in this chapter by homeopathic friend Lynne Howard who practises with me.

baby – neonatal conditions and illnesses
abdominal hernia

Description: A soft bulge or protrusion in the abdominal area, usually most apparent when the baby is crying and the stomach is hard and tense.

Explanation: This occurs when (usually a small) part of the intestine pushes through a weak spot in the muscles of the abdominal wall. Most can be classified as umbilical (around the belly button) or inguinal (around the groin area) and are more common in premature babies.

Course of action: When the baby is lying on her back and relaxed, the doctor might be able to reduce it (push the hernia back into the abdominal cavity) if the neck of the hernia is wide enough. (In general, congenital umbilical hernias may reduce and seal up on their own, and surgical intervention may not necessary.) When this is not possible – more commonly in cases of inguinal hernia – surgery is required. It is important to be aware that the abdominal hernia can sometimes get trapped. This can make the baby cry with pain or vomit.

Description: Wheezy, rattling breath; difficulty in breathing out the air rather than breathing in.

Explanation: Asthma can commonly be related to either a virus or allergy. In both instances, the child is likely to grow out of it, but boys are more affected by viral asthma and girls by allergic asthma. Viral asthma usually follows a cold and coughing, and the wheeze can hang around for months if the child quickly catches another infection. Allergic asthma often accompanies eczema and hay fever, and can also be linked to a diet allergy.

Course of action:

- Use a vaporizer in the baby's bedroom at night to keep the air moist and prevent coughing.
- Tip up the head end of the cot to help drain congestion from the airways and minimize coughing.
- If there is a heavy carpet in the baby's room, consider using a powerful vacuum cleaner that can zip away most of the dust and the mites who live in it! If at all possible, replace the heavy carpet with a hard floor like laminate, lino or wood. I have found an improvement in the chest health of babies and adults whenever carpets are replaced with hard floors.
- Keep the baby away from tobacco smoke. Refuse to remain in a room or stay in a home where people have been smoking.
- Prolonged breastfeeding – up to a year – helps protect the child from asthma (and also related eczema).
- See your GP, who may prescribe an inhaler mask (for babies) or an inhaler (for older children) for stronger attacks.
- Minimize contact with animals, particularly cats, rabbits, dogs, horses and goats.

bronchiolitis

Description: A persistent, dry cough, which becomes chesty and is accompanied by a runny nose and rapid, wheezy breathing.

Explanation: Bronchiolitis is a common viral infection which lasts for about ten to fourteen days before improving. It occurs when the bronchioles (small branches of the lungs) become inflamed and cause an over-production of mucus (mucus lines the air passages to protect the airways), leading to coughing and mild breathing difficulties.

Course of action:

- A vaporizer (with pure water only) in the baby's room will moisten the air and help her breathe more easily, so reducing coughing.
- The creative healing massage to reduce inflammation in the lungs and bronchi would be the same as the moves over the chest cage as described in the baby massage section (page 17).
- To specifically help drain the bronchi, use the tips of your index and middle finger of both your hands and gently stroke the chest downwards from the midpoint of the breastbone to a point midway between the end of the breastbone and the belly button. Perform this movement in a continuous flow with one hand following the other

for a full four minutes. Avoid using essential oils as this might
exacerbate the condition.
- Your GP may offer a nebulizer (with a mask) to administer
  medication if the baby's breathing is particularly fast or wheezy.

---

homeopathy for bronchiolitis

See the 'Coughs' section (page 246) for homeopathic indications
and remedies. I would advise seeking advice from a professional
homeopath.

---

chickenpox

See also 'Neonatal Chickenpox', page 263.

Description: Distinctive red spots – usually first appearing on the scalp
and around the hairline – rapidly multiplying to form a rash.
Explanation: The rash spots quickly turn into fluid-filled blisters and
are highly contagious – ninety-eight per cent of the adult population has
immunity because of childhood exposure. Some people even hold
'chickenpox parties' in order to get it 'over and done with'. Chickenpox
is passed by droplet exposure, such as kissing, sneezing, coughing and
sharing bottles/beakers. There is a ten- to twenty-day incubation period
before the spots appear, and the child is contagious for forty-eight hours
before the spots appear until the last of the spots has crusted over
(usually within five days). The condition often presents with a high
fever and severe itching, and the spots can cover every part of the body,
including the genitals.

Pulsatilla 30 When children are weepy, clingy with a tendency to whine, presenting with a moderate fever with little thirst, better in the open air, worse for heat and at night.

Rhus tox 30 If the eruptions are large and filled with pus, very itchy and worse from scratching, at night and when resting. There may be restlessness associated with difficulty in going to sleep.

Belladonna 30 Face is flushed and red, with very hot skin. Dilated pupils may be noted. Baby may be drowsy and unable to sleep. May twitch and start in sleep.

Mercurius 30 Indicated if you notice profuse, offensive sweat or salivation, and if the breath is offensive with the neck glands swollen. The baby feels worse by both heat and cold and at night. You may notice eruptions that form pus and may become open sores.

Ant. Tart 30 If the child is very ill-humoured. Tongue coated white. Skin rash comes out slowly. May have a rattling cough.

Arsenicum 30 Large pus-filled eruptions that may become open sores.

Mercurius 12x Burning pains better for heat or hot applications, pain and itching worse after midnight and for cold. Extreme chilliness.

Course of action:

- Scarring can occur if the spots are scratched so it's important to ease the child's itchy discomfort by keeping the spots moisturized and supple. Lacto-calamine lotion for use in the bath is preferable to just the calamine skin cream. A favourite midwife remedy is to hang a bundle of muslin filled with oats beneath the running tap; this makes the water creamy and moisturizing and is an instant soothing tonic.
- Keep the bath lukewarm, rather than hot, as a high water temperature will cause the blood vessels to dilate, making the skin more irritable.

- Cover the child's skin as much as possible (very thin layers in the summer) to prevent direct scratching and the secondary risk of infection.
- Sometimes GPs might prescribe antibiotics if there is a chest infection.
- I have found that applying pure lavender oil to the skin lesions helps reduce soreness and itching. Lavender is anti-inflammatory, antiviral and analgesic in action. Tea tree oil is known for its antiviral and antibacterial properties, but it can sting the skin on application. Instead, diffuse it by placing a few drops in a small bowl of hot water, and leave it out of reach of your baby, letting the fragrance clean the air.

clicky hips (congenital dislocation of the hips)

Description: A clicking sound/feeling which is picked up by the paediatrician at the newborn check (before discharge from hospital) and followed up at the eight-week check.

Explanation: This happens when the socket in the hipbone is too shallow to retain the 'ball' at the head of the thighbone, allowing it to slip out, or dislocate. It is more common in twins and breech babies. This can be diagnosed if one of the creases in the baby's groin is not as well defined as the other.

Course of action: If this has been identified by the paediatrician, you will be immediately referred to an orthopaedic surgeon and offered an ultrasound within six weeks of birth to see how well the ball and socket joint sit together. If the click is mild, the baby need only wear two nappies at once, instead of one, for a few weeks. Otherwise the baby will be offered a brace or plaster cast to wear for a couple of months. All treatment is usually finished by the time walking begins.

Description: Runny nose (clear to thick green), coughing (often at night), sneezing, and high temperature.

Explanation: Colds are an inevitable and necessary (immune-boosting) part of growing up. Most babies catch an average of seven colds in their first year. Most of those will occur in the latter six months, when the natural immunity they were born with has depleted, although prolonged breastfeeding will boost this as the baby will continue to receive your antibodies and therefore protection from the illnesses going around. Premature babies are more prone to coughs and colds as their immune systems are more immature. Most infections are viral and disappear within three to four days but can turn into a bacterial infection if there is no improvement after this point. Signs of this change include a consistently high temperature, lack of appetite and a chesty cough.

Course of action:

- Colds are often worse at night when the baby is lying on her back and nasal passages become more congested. An electric vaporizer can make it much easier for the baby to breathe and can stay on for most of the night (around ten hours, so turn it on when you go to bed).

- A traditional eucalyptus chest rub (a very gentle rub!) is also effective. For this, mix just two drops of pure organic eucalyptus oil in two teaspoons of virgin olive oil. Then perform the creative healing method of drainage massage on the chest as described in the general baby massage section (page 17).

- For little babies under three months, put some drops of pure organic eucalyptus oil onto a muslin cloth knot-tied to the baby's cot, or drop a couple of drops onto their sleep suit on the upper part near their chest area.

- Prop up the head end of the baby's cot on small castors to help drain the nasal passages and reduce night-time coughing. The Mouche-Bébé (see page 19) is a great help to drain the anterior nasal passages and make the baby more comfortable. You could also use a couple of nose drops of pure saline to make the mucus runny and therefore easier for the baby to clear away. (Saline nose drops for babies can be purchased from a chemist.)

- If the baby has a temperature, offer 2.5–5ml of infant paracetamol once every eight hours for about three days, or until the fever subsides. (There are links between ibuprofen and childhood asthma and stomach complaints, so do not give this to your baby.)
- If the infection is bacterial, antibiotics will clear it up quickly.

Cautionary note: Echinacea is often suggested as an immune-boost for adults when a flu or a cold hits them but is not suitable for children under three years of age.

---

creative healing for colds

Carry out a sinus-drainage treatment along the maxillary sinus areas. If there is an accompanying chest infection, a lung-drainage treatment can be applied.

Method: Place your fingertips very lightly over the nose, exactly where the soft nasal cartilage ends and the fleshy part begins. Then very gently make two tiny circular movements, with the intention of opening the drainage pathways, and then draw the fingertips of each hand down and away from the nostril, tracing a line below the cheekbones on either side as you draw your fingertips up towards the front of the ear (to the dip just above the triangular flap, the tragus) in front of the ear.

Homeopathy for Colds

Ferrum Phos 30 Give during the first stage of inflammation when there are no clear symptoms but a slight fever.

Aconite 30 Can be given for the first stage of illness, for symptoms that come on suddenly after exposure to a cold, dry wind. There may be frequent sneezing, burning throat, thirst, hot, and restlessness at night.

Belladonna 30 Symptoms come on suddenly, such as after exposing the head to cold or washing the hair. The face is flushed and the skin feels hot and dry. The sore throat is often bright red, worse on the right side. There maybe restlessness and sensitivity to light. There is a fever, and the head may be hot with cold extremities. Pupils are dilated and the baby is generally worse at night.

Bryonia 30 When the child wants to be left alone and to lie still, and is worse from the slightest movement. The baby may be thirsty or hungry. Cold tends to travel into the chest. Lips and mouth are dry. There may be a watery discharge and a stuffy nose.

Dulcamara 30 When there has been a sudden onset of symptoms from a change of weather, such as from hot to cold. There is profuse watery discharge from the nose and eyes. You may notice that the nose runs more in a warm room.

Pulsatilla 30 Thick, creamy, bland mucus. The child is worse for warmth and desires, and is better for, fresh air. The child could be thirstless, weepy and clingy and exhibit a changeable nature.

Natrum Mur 30 Clear nasal discharge that looks like egg white. Could have an associated loss of smell and taste. Sneezing can be observed in early stages. May have watery discharge from eyes.

Hepar Sulp Lots of thick, yellow mucus causing a rattling sound. Irritable and sweaty. Better for damp weather and worse in dry, cold weather.

Arsenicum Album 30 Clear, burning discharge from nose. Anxious and restless. Worse after midnight. Burning pains that are relieved by heat.

Gelsemium 30 Slow onset. Lethargic, heavy eyed, chilly with dull headache. Much sneezing and watery discharge. Thirstless. Muscles may ache.

Nux Vomica 30 Early stages of a cold. Sneezing, nose runny during the day and blocked up at night. Sore throat. The baby feels cold, is worse in the cold air and irritable.

Mercurius 30 Chilliness and sneezing. Either thick, yellow-green nasal discharge or profuse watery discharge irritates the nose and upper lip. Foul breath, perhaps a metallic taste. The baby may smell of vomit.

See 'Coughs' for further relevant information.

colic

Description: Inconsolable crying, diagnosed according to the rule of threes: coming on at about three weeks, generally lasting for at least three hours a day, at least three days a week, for at least three weeks. During an attack the baby will mostly draw her legs up to the tummy or straighten them out rigidly, sometimes kicking out and shrieking with pain. It is usually gone by three months, but can take up to six months to resolve.

Explanation: Infant colic has been linked to formula-fed babies and to babies whose mothers smoked during pregnancy, specifically during the first four months. The exact cause is not known and even the symptoms are erratic – some babies cry in episodes, others non-stop; generally the attacks come on in the early evening but they can occur earlier. Explanations range from an immature gut which goes into spasm and contracts painfully to a distressing or protracted birth that has compressed the cranium and the cranial base and disturbed the neural pathways leading to the digestive tract. For breastfeeding babies, reasons for colic are thought to include a poor latch with associated swallowing of air; and a sudden change in the mother's diet, or certain foods/drinks in her diet that pass into the breast milk and irritate the baby's stomach. For formula-fed babies, culprits can be a sensitivity to cow's milk or swallowing too much air during a feed. It has been found that in babies with infant colic, all three gut hormones are raised (motilin, gastrin and VIP (vaso active intestinal peptide).

Course of action:

- Cranial osteopathy should be the first course of action, particularly following an instrumental or long, difficult birth. Find a practitioner who works a lot with newborns or small babies (see Resources). One appointment with a follow-up session is usual.
- Body contact is key. Even for those babies for whom nothing really works, just holding the baby provides a level of comfort, even if the episode persists. Of course, it is difficult for the parent to be so close to the screaming infant, but this dynamic, sympathetic parenting will help forge a close long-term bond.
- Keeping the baby upright (perhaps in a sling) can be useful. Some mothers swear by pacing up and down the stairs. Others say the Tiger in the Tree position (see page 77) often soothes the baby during an attack.
- Midwives often swear by fennel tea for soothing colicky babies. Fennel tea for babies is made by adding a quarter teaspoon of fennel seeds to 100ml of filtered water in an enamel saucepan – bring to the boil and then allow to simmer for ten minutes. Then strain and cool to room temperature. Give a teaspoon of this decoction to the baby five minutes before and after feeds. The baby will only need about four to six teaspoons a day, and the mother can drink the leftover fennel tea.
- Alternatively, try a drop of Infacol before each feed, or a spoonful of gripe water immediately after. These work by merging and enlarging the air bubbles in the tummy, making it easier for the baby to burp them back up.
- A warm aromatherapy bath may help calm her down. Add two drops of lavender essential oil to the water, together with two drops of fennel or anise. There is no doubt that the skin is very absorbent.

Essential oil baths allow the medicinal properties of the essential oils to manifest rather quickly. Both fennel and anise are known to release bowel spasm. Make sure you hold your baby securely in her little bath.

- Massage isn't advisable during an attack as the baby's tummy is likely to be hard and tender, but it can be applied before as a deterrent and afterwards as a balm on an ongoing 'maintenance' basis. The 'I love you' triangle (firm strokes starting from the pubic bone, up to the baby's left hip, across to the right and back down to the pubic bone) is good, as are cycling the legs and Ayurvedic leg stretches (see page 19).

---

homeopathy for colic

Homeopathy can be very effective in treating colic. Give one dose each bedtime for five days.

Mag Phos 30 Passing wind or belching may not help. Persistent hiccup with retching may occur. Better for pressure, heat and doubling up.

Colocynthis 30 More of an angry baby, more restless and irritable than the Mag Phos. type. Tongue may be coated. Better for pressure, heat and doubling up.

Chamomilla 30 Doubles up and screams with a hot, flushed face and sweat. Irritable. Better for heat and being carried. Symptoms are worse at night; there is green diarrhoea associated with a smell of rotten eggs.

Dioscorea 30 For sudden colic. Worse for doubling up, better for stretching out, better with heat and firm pressure.

---

effective winding

Make sure to wind the baby effectively after each feed (see also page 59) to eliminate air bubbles in the tummy. These can be uncomfortable if they pass into the intestine as trapped wind.

If you are breastfeeding:
- Eliminate 'windy' foods such as peas, beans, lentils, onions, cabbage, cauliflower, broccoli and sprouts.
- Avoid alcohol, caffeine and spicy foods.
- Eat an optimum diet so that you and, through your milk, your baby get all the nutrients you need. Avoid skipping meals.
- Drink two litres of filtered or purified water each day.
- Mothers can also drink nettle tea as it is a good liver detoxer and might help cleanse the mother's circulating plasma volume and help clarify the milk.

If your baby is bottle-fed:
- Try switching teats – from a 0 to 1 if the baby is impatient and restless and sucking lots of air on the bottle, or go down a level if the baby seems to struggle with the milk flow and is gulping for air. Alternatively, try XX Brown bottles. These have a special teat and bottle specifically designed for soothing colic.
- Look for a brand of formula milk that contains probiotics (the natural enzymes already found in the baby's gut) and enzymes (similar to the enzymes of the milk curds that make it easier for the baby to digest and may help reduce indigestion).

conjunctivitis ('sticky eye')

Description: Yellow/whitish pus oozing from the inner corners of the eye; eyelids stuck together or crusty eyelashes upon waking; or eye feels gritty, red and sore.

Explanation: Bacterial conjunctivitis is the most common form of this eye infection and is contagious. Lots of discharge is produced and it's important to try to keep the baby from rubbing her eyes, getting it on her hands and spreading it further. Viral conjunctivitis feels more like something is in your eye, inducing lots of rubbing, but it can also have some pus discharge.

Course of action:

- Wipe the eyes first thing in the morning with cotton wool dipped in boiled water. Always sweep from the inner corner to out, using a new piece of cotton wool each time. Never reuse a piece of cotton as you risk reinfecting the eye.
- Avoid sharing towels or clothes (such as jumpers and T-shirts).
- Try to keep siblings and other family members from cheek-to-cheek contact.
- You can buy over-the-counter antibacterial drops from your pharmacist.
- If the amount of discharge increases or changes from white to yellow, see your GP to get a prescription for local antibiotic drops (if the infection is bacterial).
- When administering to babies and small children, it's easier to use eye drops. These are increasingly being replaced by water-soluble viscose gels. Squeeze a drop onto the inner corners of the eye, even if their eyes are closed. Stop them from rubbing their eyes and encourage them to look at you so that the drops fall into the eyelid and spread out to the rest of the conjunctiva.
- If your child sleeps very heavily, you can try applying the drops or ointment while she is sleeping.

constipation

Description: Difficulty, inability or no urge to pass stools after three or more days. Stools are hard, solid and formed.

Explanation: Slightly different to the causes in adults, there are huge swings between what can be considered constipation in one child, and not in another. Some babies poo several times a day (even several times a feed!) while others can go for up to a week without opening their bowels. Breastfeeding promotes optimum production of the hormone motilin within the baby's gut, which aids peristalsis (the muscular movements in the bowel wall that move the contents along). Formula-fed babies are more likely to suffer from constipation as the manufactured milk is thicker, harder to digest and contains no motilin. When babies are weaned, diet and drinking should be closely monitored to make sure enough fibre is being ingested so that stools are soft and easy to push out.

Course of action:

- If you are breastfeeding, make sure you drink at least two litres of water a day to ensure your milk hydrates the baby.
- For bottle-fed babies, supplement with a bottle of cool, boiled water for baby to sip throughout the day. Keep a bottle next to the cot to offer at night-time wakings once the baby has dropped the nightly milk feeds.
- For bottle-fed babies, make sure you are mixing enough water with the powder. Use a scoop, level off each one before putting it in the water and do not make guesstimates.

- When weaning, get into the habit of offering water at regular intervals through the day, not just at mealtimes.
- Be careful with bananas. You should offer only very ripe bananas mashed with overcooked rice or porridge with a handful of raisins or prunes on top.
- For toddlers, a little box of raisins, dried apricots or prunes will quickly become a favourite snack and protect against constipation.
- Warm baths can help the baby's tummy relax, which will help.
- Post-bath massage (the 'I love you' triangle and cycling legs movements, see page 241) will encourage movement in the bowels.
- Cranial osteopathy is successful in treating prolonged constipation.
- Daily reflexology massages on the soles of the tiny baby's feet have been known to stimulate the colon reflexes and keep the bowels regular.
- A seven-minute, creative healing, light-touch massage on the dimples of the sacrum is very effective (see page 93). To gauge pressure, be sure not to leave any redness on the skin.
- Colourlight therapy offers a very effective treatment of applying pinpoints of coloured light to the abdomen to treat constipation – quick, easy and effective! (See Resources.)
- Attitudes to pooing can have a considerable effect, even on little babies. Make sure it is not referred to as dirty or laughed at, and try to praise – rather than roll your eyes at – each movement. Do not refer to the smell or look away when changing nappies. Remember, it's better out than in!

Cautionary note: Very rarely, prolonged and/or severe constipation can be symptomatic of a more serious physical condition. For instance, there can be varying degrees of Hirschsprung's disease where there is an actual congenital lack in the development of nerve ganglia in the bowel wall; or there may be a bowel obstruction. See your GP if constipation is not resolved within a week of trying the above treatments.

Alumen 30 Stool dry and hard, large or like sheep's dung. No desire to evacuate for several days.

Alumina 30 Great straining, even for a soft stool. Stools are hard and knotty, or soft and clayey, adhering to skin. Worse from artificial food.

Silica 30 Extremely hard and large stools. Strains, but the stool recedes back into the rectum after being partly expelled.

Plumbum Met 30 Stools hard, lumpy and black-brown like sheep's dung. Child cries in agony while attempting to pass a stool.

Lycopodium 6c Stools are hard and knotty. Flatulence. Ineffectual desire to pass stool. Worse between 4pm and 8pm. Eating even a little produces a sense of fullness.

Calc Carb 30 The stool is at first hard, then pasty and then liquid and of a light colour.

Bryonia 30 Stool is large, hard and dry, dark as if burnt. Stools are passed with great difficulty Irritability.

See 'Constipation' in the mother's section for more remedies and symptoms.

homeopathy for coughs

Here are some of the main remedies used in treating coughs, but there are many more. Consult a homeopath if the cough does not improve or if it doesn't fit one of the following descriptions:

Aconite See the 'Croup' section for symptoms.

Antimonium Tart 30 For loose, coarse, rattling cough, but with scanty expectoration. May have suffocating shortness of breath. Worse for warmth and in the evening.

Belladonna 30 If red-faced, burning hot with dilated pupils. Sudden onset can present as a dry, teasing cough. Worse at night.

Bryonia 30 For a dry, painful cough. Worse on entering a warm room and with movement. Thirst for cold drinks.

Chamomilla 30 Dry, tickling, irritating cough, worse at night but doesn't wake the child who may be irritable and capricious. Worse during teething. Better for being carried.

Drosera 30 Violent, spasmodic cough, deep, barking, hollow, may end in gagging and/or vomiting. Whooping cough. Worse after midnight.

Hepar Sulp 30 See the 'Croup' section for symptoms.

Ipecac 30 Dry, spasmodic cough, ending in choking, gagging and vomiting.

Kali Bic 30 Brassy and hacking sound that seems to come from a tickle in the larynx. With sputum that is stringy and yellow.

Phos 30 Cough dry, tickling or hacking with hoarseness and loss of voice. Burning pain in chest. Thirsty. Worse for change of weather, cold air, during the morning after getting up. Better for heat.

Pulsatilla 30 Dry cough in the evening but sounds loose in the morning. May be gagging and choking and bringing up thick yellow-green mucus. Worse for becoming warm in bed and lying down. Better for sitting up and open air. Clingy, whiny and weepy.

Spongia 30 See the 'Croup' section for symptoms.

coughs

Explanation: Coughs normally follow on from a cold, or a residual chest infection is left after general flu-like symptoms. A cough can be caused by a virus, and this generally develops into bronchiolitis (see page 231). Sometimes this can progress to pneumonia if left untreated (see page 264).

Course of action: Commonly, coughs can be treated with homeopathy and simple cough linctus. If a cough lasts for more than two weeks and is tending to get chesty, a GP would prescribe antibiotics, but only if the cough is accompanied by green sputum, indicating a secondary bacterial infection. The General Medical Council has a directive that antibiotics are not to be used on babies and children as a first-line treatment for coughs.

cradle cap

Description: A crusted mass of thick, yellowy, scaly skin covering areas of the scalp.

Explanation: Cradle cap is a form of eczema which is very common in newborns and young children. It is not uncomfortable or itchy, and occurs when the sebaceous glands are overproductive and the skin on the scalp gets firm and hard.

Course of action:

- There are plenty of over-the-counter specialist shampoos – such as Dentinox – which tackle cradle cap. The response is usually rapid – within two to three washes.
- Alternatively, mix a couple of drops of lavender and/or tea tree oil with a good base oil such as extra virgin olive oil or fine almond oil, and rhythmically massage the scalp. Be gentle while massaging around the fontanelle.
- Avoid picking at the scaly skin as this poses the risk of infection.

Description: Rattled breathing accompanied by a sharp, high, barking cough.

Explanation: Croup is a respiratory infection which sometimes occurs after a cold and is particularly bad at night. The virus affects the larynx and chest area, which react by producing mucus, thereby narrowing the airways. It can sound more serious than it actually is but your child may become frightened by the sounds she is making, so it's important to soothe her. Breathing may sound particularly laboured (especially under three years) as the airways are inflamed, but revert to the first rule of first aid and check that her airways are clear.

Course of action:

- Try to calm her with some steam inhalations. With babies and small children, sit on the toilet with them on your lap and run the hot water in the shower/bath (or both), keeping the door shut. (Open the window after ten minutes or so.) The steam should loosen the mucus congestion, making breathing easier.
- If the child is older, place some steaming water in a bowl and bend the child's head over it, with a towel over the head to trap the steam. If there is no improvement after fifteen minutes, seek emergency medical help.
- If the steam does work, give the baby some milk or water, as their throat may be dry and sore, before returning to bed.
- A vaporizer with just pure water will help humidify the air and keep it moist. It might be best to avoid essential oils as the mucus membranes could be sensitive, and this could set off another attack.

Cautionary note: Urgent medical attention is required if the baby is too breathless to take the breast or bottle; if her breath is drawing in the stomach deeply and sharply beneath the ribcage; if she is struggling to breathe, even when calm. Epiglottitis is a throat infection which shares many of the symptoms of croup. It also includes drooling and jutting the lower jaw forward. Although it is very rare, it is something to be aware of, as it can lead to meningitis.

homeopathy for croup

The first remedies to consider for croup are Aconite, Hepar Sulp and Spongia. If these are not indicated, refer to the 'Cough' section for more ideas.

Aconite 30 First stages of inflammation. Comes on suddenly after exposure to cold, dry wind. Constant short, dry, barking cough, wakes the baby from sleep. Worse on entering a warm room, at night and in cold, dry air.

Hepar Sulp 30 Loose, rattling and croupy cough. Lots of mucus, which is sticky, thick and yellow. Cough is barking, hacking, loose in the morning and dry at night. Worse after exposure to cold, dry wind, in the early morning, before midnight and for being uncovered. Better for warmth.

Spongia 30 Cough sounds hollow, barking, crowing, sawing, croupy. Mucous membranes are dry. Worse for cold, dry wind, cold drinks, exertion and when roused from sleep. Better for eating warm food and drinks.

diarrhoea

Description: Loose, watery stools; a sudden increase in the number and amount of stools passed.

Explanation: Usually stemming from an infection, the baby is contagious for a couple of days before onset and whilst it persists. The germs can be transmitted through touch so washing your hands after each nappy change and before feeding is vital. Also make sure the baby does not put her hands down to the genitals whilst you are changing the nappy. If diarrhoea continues beyond twenty-four hours, dehydration becomes a concern (exacerbated if accompanied by vomiting, sweating or a streaming nose). Signs of dehydration include dry nappies, very yellow urine, dry lips, listlessness and a sunken fontanelle. Severe dehydration (classified as loss of fifteen per cent body weight) requires immediate hospitalization for intravenous fluid and electrolyte replacement.

Course of action:

- If diarrhoea is severe or prolonged or you suspect dehydration, go immediately to your doctor, taking your baby's red book with you so that her history of weight gain can be accurately noted.

- If you are breastfeeding then keep feeding – this provides fluids, nutrients and anti-infective agents to help cure the baby. Feed more often than usual.

- Where diarrhoea is accompanied with vomiting, cease formula milk feeds (but continue breast milk feeds) for twelve to twenty-four hours. (Dehydration, not starvation, is the immediate concern.) Formula-fed infants should be constantly offered sips of cool, boiled water. Little and often is better than bursts of gulping (particularly if there is vomiting as well).

- If your baby is weaned, dramatically cut back the diet to just fluids. Once the baby easily keeps down fluids without retching or vomiting, reintroduce plain foods such as baby rice and maybe wheat-free baby rusks and apple purée.

- Buy a rehydration treatment such as paediatric Diarolyte from your chemist. This contains electrolytes which are normally lost in the diarrhoea. Give the fluids in a sterilized bottle, beaker or even as teaspoons, depending on how young the child is and if there is vomiting. You can give Diarolyte to both breast- and formula-fed infants.
- A simple, low-cost electrolyte replacement that my father used to prescribe in his paediatric practice in India was to take a glass of boiled and cooled water and add two teaspoons of sugar, two pinches of sea salt (sodium chloride) and half a teaspoon of lime or lemon juice. Mix well and put into a sterilized feeding bottle. Make more of this solution to rehydrate the baby for two to three days and till the diarrhoea has resolved. Of course, a doctor will have to monitor the progress of the baby all the way till recovery.
- Change dirty nappies immediately as the urine will be very strong and cause severe nappy rash if left too long.
- After each nappy change, apply a protective barrier cream. I particularly like the calendula nappy cream from Weleda. You could take your pick from the vast variety of organic baby lotions that are flooding the market now. Try to avoid products containing petroleum.
- Avoid very sweet fruit juices or dairy products as they can aggravate the diarrhoea. Sugary substances increase the bacterial count in the intestines.

homeopathy for diarrhoea

Here are some of the main remedies used in treating diarrhoea, but there are many more. Consult a homeopath if the diarrhoea does not improve or if it does not fit one of the following descriptions.

Aconite 30 Sudden onset of attack. Severe pain noted before and during stool. Occurs after exposure to cold or during summer. Could occur after fright. Stools might look green like chopped spinach.

Aethusa 30 If you have noticed an inability to digest milk. Frequently indicated for diarrhoea during dentition. Diarrhoea is light-yellow.

Arsenicum Album 30 When you notice associated restlessness with thirst. Stools are watery, brownish, copious and foul-smelling. Symptoms are worse after midnight. Anxiety noticed. Give if you think diarrhoea is a result of eating spoilt food.

Belladonna 30 Face and eyes are red and the hands are hot during fever. Baby starts suddenly from sleep, as if frightened. You can give this if diarrhoea occurs during teething. Stools are thin, green and with lumps like chalk. Summer diarrhoea.

Chamomilla 30 If irritable and impatient, and when diarrhoea occurs during teething. Stools are hot, green, watery, fetid and slimy. White and yellow mucus pieces are often noted in stools.

Podophyllum 30 If occurs during teething or hot weather or after acid fruits. Stools are green, watery, fetid, profuse and gushing. Baby passes stool with big noise owing to accumulated wind. Worse early in the morning.

Pulsatilla 30 Stools are changeable. May be associated with nausea, griping, belching and thirstlessness. Weepy, clingy child.

ear infection

Description: Redness in the ear. The baby rubs or pulls on the ear or shakes her head. Cheek pain or pain when sucking. White or yellow pus oozing from the ear.

---

homeopathy for ear infection

Chronic otitis media (commonly called glue ear) is believed to arise out of a fundamental weakness in the child's constitution or from suppressive therapeutic intervention such as antibiotic treatment, and needs to be treated by a homeopath. Here are some of the main remedies for acute ear infection:

Aconite 30 Sudden onset, following exposure to a cold, dry wind. Symptoms include fever, thirst, dryness. Gets worse with noise, covering and in a warm room.

Belladonna 30 If there is a sudden onset there will be intense throbbing and burning pain. The baby becomes bright red with a dry, intense fever. Pupils are dilated. Symptoms are worse at night. Baby favours the right side.

Pulsatilla 30 Baby is weepy, clingy, whiny and thirstless. Discharge is thick, yellow-green, bland and purulent. Symptoms are worse in the evening and night and with heat.

Chamomilla 30 Baby is irritable and capricious. The emotional state often leads to this presciption. Symptoms are worse at 9am and 9pm, and in the cold air; better for heat and being carried.

Lycopodium 30 Worse on the right side or right moving to left side. Symptoms are worse between 4pm and 8pm. Baby may be flatulent with a dry cough, and can have eczema around and behind the ear.

Mercurius 30 Foul breath, increased salivation and flabby tongue. Profuse, offensive perspiration. Symptoms are worse at night. Can have green discharge. Favours the right side.

Explanation: Most commonly, an infection in the middle ear that fills with mucus and leads to a steady build-up of tension and pain. In extreme cases, this can lead to the eardrum rupturing.

Course of action:

- Ask your doctor to examine the baby's ears. Never use cotton buds to try to clean or investigate the eardrum yourself.
- Infant paracetamol will bring down an associated high temperature.
- Lots of cuddles and body contact will soothe and reassure the baby.
- About a third of all ear infections originate from a food allergy, so try eliminating cow's milk from your baby's diet (dairy products have been associated with increased mucus production).
- If there is no improvement after three days, your doctor may prescribe antibiotics.

eczema

Description: A raised red rash or cluster of small spots, usually found on the arms, upper legs, trunk and face.

Explanation: Eczema is an inflammation of the skin which causes itching or a burning feeling. It is very common, not contagious and does not scar. Most children grow out of the condition and it can be easily treated. Quite often, the condition is worse in the cold winter months and clears up during the summer.

Course of action:

- Add an emollient – such as Oilatum – to the baby's bath water to help keep the skin moisturized and supple. (You may need to shop around for one that suits your baby best, as some skins can be sensitive to their ingredients.)
- Aqueous creams – such as Diprobase – can make a dramatic difference if applied daily after baths and at nappy changes.
- Avoid using soap, which can be drying.
- Antihistamines – such as Piriton syrup – can help reduce itchiness.

- If the skin is scratched and becomes infected, an antiseptic cream may be required.
- If the eczema becomes angry and inflamed, your GP will prescribe a topical steroid cream.
- Use the mildest washing powder you can and make sure it is non-biological (I like the Fairy or Ecover brands) or wash with pure water only.

---

homeopathy for eczema

Eczema needs to be treated by a homeopath as many remedies are used to treat this condition, and courses of treatment depend on the overall health of the patient. During treatment there can sometimes be an aggravation of symptoms, which needs to be managed by a professional homeopath.

---

fractured collarbone

Description: Fracture of one or both sides of the collarbone during birth.

Explanation: This is most common when the baby is too large, or the mother's pelvis too small, and it is difficult to deliver the baby's shoulders. The collarbone is placed under severe pressure as the shoulders squeeze through, resulting in a greenstick fracture. It will be apparent there is a bone injury if the baby cries upon being picked up (when the ribcage is compressed, thereby putting pressure on the collarbone) or if the baby is not moving one or both arms.

Course of action: Babies' bones knit together incredibly quickly, and the fracture will heal within seven to ten days. For older children, a sling is advised for immobilizing the arm, but this presents a suffocation risk to wriggly little babies, so most doctors advise pinning the sleeve of the sleep suit onto the middle section at the front.

---

homeopathy for a fractured collarbone

Arnica 30 will help with bruising and shock. If the bone is slow to heal or extremely painful, consult a homeopath as there are several remedies that can be used to ease pain and speed the recovery from broken bones.

---

gastroenteritis

Description: Projectile vomiting; severe diarrhoea; listlessness; fever; loss of appetite; stomach pain.

Explanation: Gastroenteritis is a relatively common viral infection (it could also be bacterial) which inflames the lining of the gut. It usually passes within a week but sometimes disappears only to flare up again, as much as six weeks later.

Course of action:

- If you are breastfeeding, keep going – feed more frequently to provide fluid, nutrition and antibodies.
- Stop formula feeds for at least twenty-four hours, or until the baby can tolerate heavier feeds. Keep the baby hydrated with plenty of sips of cool, boiled water.
- If the vomiting and diarrhoea persist beyond forty-eight hours, use an electrolyte solution –such as Diarolyte – to keep the baby from becoming dehydrated (breast- and formula-fed babies).
- Encourage lots of bed rest.
- Keep your hands scrupulously clean after nappy changes and before preparing food, to avoid reinfecting the baby.

- Make sure the baby does not touch his bottom or genitals during nappy changes, to prevent reinfection.
- Change the baby out of dirty nappies immediately to prevent a sore case of nappy rash.
- In severe gastroenteritis, it is good medical policy to send a sample of stool to the microbiologist. If the microbiologist detects a virulent bug then the appropriate antibiotic can be prescribed.

homeopathy for gastroenteritis

China 12x China can be used to rehydrate the baby when there is dehydration because of loss of fluids, with weakness and exhaustion.

Arsenicum Album 30 Acute vomiting and diarrhoea after food poisoning. The baby vomits bile. Other symptoms include fainting and sweating after vomiting, sweating while vomiting and burning pains after passing a stool. Stools are smelly and watery. Baby is restless and anxious. Symptoms are worse after midnight.

Veratrum Album 30 Baby alternates between vomiting and diarrhoea. Has a cold sweat, especially on forehead.

Phosphorus 30 Baby vomits food or drink as soon as it becomes warm in the stomach. There is burning and soreness in the stomach. Baby vomits bile and is thirsty.

Ipecac 30 Nausea, griping pains in intestines, with or without vomiting. Clean tongue. Nausea worse for looking at moving objects.

Colocynthis 30 Severe pain causes doubling up. Better for pressure and warmth to stomach.

Antimonium Crudum 30 Vomiting caused by overeating or eating some indigestible substance. Vomits soon after eating or drinking. Tongue coated white.

Description: Yellowing of the skin or whites of the eyes; excessive sleepiness.

Explanation: Jaundice arises in the first few days after birth when the baby's immature liver cannot break down the foetal haemoglobin quickly enough (which the baby needed in the womb). As the foetal haemoglobin breaks down, it produces a yellow pigment called bilirubin. If produced more quickly than it can be excreted, it is deposited in the skin. Jaundice is a common condition, affecting sixty per cent of babies (particularly Caucasians), and is more prevalent in premature babies, or those with moderate to severe bruising following a long, hard or instrumental birth. It is rarely serious but, if left unchecked, risks the bilirubin crossing over into the brain and causing brain damage.

Course of action:

- Regular feeds every three hours during the day and every four hours at night will help to break down and digest the bilirubin levels.
- The more severe the jaundice, the more sleepy the baby, so it is even more important to wake the baby for feeds and not wait for her to ask.
- Place the baby in sunlight as much as possible and expose the skin as much as the temperature allows. If it is too cold to go outside, just place the baby to sleep and/or play on a mat by a bright window.
- If the baby is yellow and losing or not gaining weight, despite frequent feeds, see your GP.
- If after two or three days the baby stays yellowish, see your GP for a blood test.
- If the bilirubin levels are above the level on the chart, phototherapy may be required in hospital.
- In very rare cases with severe jaundice, phototherapy is not successful and a blood transfusion may be required.

measles

Description: A raised rash, often first appearing behind the ears, accompanied by a cough and fever, and sometimes an eye infection.

Explanation: Contagious from two days before the rash appears and until four days afterwards, measles is spread by droplets – sneezing, coughing, kissing and sharing bottles etc. It is relatively rare these days due to the early vaccination age, although the controversy surrounding the MMR jab (which is supposed to protect against measles, mumps and rubella) has led to a lower take-up in some areas, giving rise to fears of outbreaks and epidemics. In the worst cases, consequences from measles include pneumonia, deafness, encephalitis and brain damage.

Course of action:

- Treat the high temperature immediately with infant paracetamol and go to see your doctor. They will take a saliva swab or blood test to check for measles antibodies.
- Drink lots of fluids and encourage bed rest.

There are many homeopathic remedies for measles, including the following:

Ferrum Phos 30 May be given at the beginning of illness when there are few symptoms but a fever developing.

Aconite 30 Restlessness; eyes ache in the light; eyes and nose streaming; a hard, croupy cough. Useful in the early stages.

Pulsatilla 30 Cough dry at night, loose in the daytime. Worse at dusk. Baby is weepy, whiny and clingy. Symptoms are worse for heat and better for fresh air.

Belladonna 30 Baby is restless, flushed and thirstless. Sore throat, and bothered by noise, light and jarring.

Gelsemium 30 Aching pains; lethargic and drowsy; headache; chilly though feverish; harsh cough and nasal discharge that irritates the nose and upper lip.

Bryonia 30 Where the rash slow to develop, Bryonia can help bring the rash out and relieve symptoms. Cough is dry and painful and worse for motion. Thirst for large amounts of cold water at long intervals.

Euphrasia 30 Eyes are sensitive to light, red and swollen with acrid tears that irritate the cheeks. There is a bland nasal discharge and a harsh cough.

meningitis

Description: Stiff neck; rash that does not fade under pressure; headache; sensitivity to light; vomiting; fever; listlessness; a high-pitched, pained cry; bulging fontanelles; bluish-tinged skin; head and neck arched backwards.
Explanation: This is when the meninges (lining of the brain) become infected, causing inflammation and a build-up of the fluids which

protect the brain. Most often, meningitis is viral, not serious and passes quickly, but there are handfuls of more severe cases in which the side-effects are long-term. Bacterial meningitis is much rarer but also more serious, leading in the worst instances to deafness, fits and brain damage. Symptoms often come on very quickly and are, unfortunately, similar to many other common childhood illnesses. The glass test for rashes is the most reliable indicator to get immediate medical help, but see a doctor straight away if your baby presents any of the above symptoms. To do the glass test, roll a clear drinking glass on the skin. If the rash remains then this could be an indication of meningitis, and the condition merits investigation in hospital.

Course of action: Seek **immediate** professional medical help. If meningitis is suspected, your baby will be put on antibiotics immediately, even if the infection turns out to be viral, as the results from the bacterial tests take forty-eight hours. **It is important to act quickly.**

mumps

Description: Swollen cheeks and neck; difficulty swallowing; dry mouth; fever.

Explanation: A viral infection which causes the cheek's salivary glands to swell, it is spread by exposure to saliva droplets, such as sneezing, coughing, kissing or sharing bottles. The child is infectious for a six-day incubation period before the swelling comes up and for ten to fourteen days afterwards. Most people recover without long-term effects, although approximately one in twenty-five suffers deafness, which is partially or fully resolved within a few weeks. Serious complications can include inflammation of the pancreas and even meningitis. As well as posing a threat to small, un-immunized children, mumps also has repercussions across all age groups – it can lead to miscarriage in pregnant women, and swollen testicles and compromised fertility in young men.

homeopathy for mumps

Belladonna 30 Rapid onset; high fever; great redness; dilated pupils; hot head and cold extremities; especially affects the right side; dryness and burning in the throat, with shooting pains in the glands; throbbing pains.

Phytolacca 30 Parotid and submandibular glands swollen and inflamed; may be stony hard. Pains often shoot into the ears on swallowing. Symptoms are generally worse for cold, wet weather, at night, and the heat of the bed. Phytolacca may also be needed if the breast, ovaries or testicles become affected.

Pulsatilla 30 Often indicated if it lingers, in the later stages. Child is weepy and clingy; desires open air and worse for heat. Thirstless with tongue coated yellow or white. Symptoms are worse at night and when lying down. The testes or breasts may be inflamed.

Apis 30 Face puffy; swollen eyelids; red oedematous swellings; burning and stinging pains. Very sensitive to touch and pressure. Symptoms are worse for heat.

Jaborandi 30 Profuse saliva, resembling egg white; dry mouth and intense thirst. Swelling of the tonsils; stiff jaw; profuse sweat.

Mercurius 30 Profuse sweat and salivation with offensive odour; sweating much more at night. Metallic taste in the mouth. Especially affects the right side.

Lycopodium 30 Swelling moves from right side to the left. Feels better from and desires warm drinks.

Lachesis 30 Swollen parotid gland, especially on the left side. Sensitive to the least touch or pressure.

Bryonia 30 Slightest motion causes pain. Baby is irritable and wants to be left alone. Much thirst for cold water.

Rhus tox 30 Baby is restless, chilly and sensitive to cold. There is swelling on the left and then the right side. Cold sores on the lips. Worse for cold, cold winds and cold, wet weather.

Course of action:

- Vaccination against mumps at thirteen months with the MMR vaccine is supposed to protect against measles, mumps and rubella, but controversy surrounding the jab has led to a dramatic fall in take-up in certain areas.
- If your child gets mumps before her vaccination, use infant paracetamol to reduce fever, and see your GP.
- Give lots of fluids to soothe the mouth.
- Warm wet towels wrapped around the cheeks can provide relief from the pain.

neonatal chickenpox

Description: Chickenpox which occurs in babies fewer than twenty-one days old, or born to mothers who develop a rash in the last five days of pregnancy.

Explanation: Extremely rare, but as with standard chickenpox, an irritating, itchy rash of fluid-filled blisters. The lesions are highly contagious until the spots crust over (see 'Chickenpox'). It must be treated medically as complications can include deafness and brain damage.

Course of action: If the mother is exposed in the last few days of her pregnancy, she can be given an immuno-globulin injection to boost her immunity and help lessen the severity of the infection. The baby will be given a VZIG antibody injection at birth.

pneumonia

Description: Listlessness, accompanied by rapid, laboured breathing which can lead to blue lips and nails. Fever is common, as is chest pain.

Explanation: Pneumonia can be bacterial or viral. Viral pneumonia is infectious but passes quickly. Viral pneumonia could originate from a cold from which the child is not recovering. Bacterial pneumonia can creep in as a secondary infection following a viral chest infection. Pnemococcal pneumonia is a common cause of serious bacterial pneumonia.

Course of action:

- If your baby has a high spiking temperature and cold, clammy skin, together with episodes of sweating profusely and struggling for breath, go straight to your GP (during the day). Your GP will then refer your baby as an emergency to your closest paediatric unit for admission and treatment.
- If your baby needs attention after office hours, phone your GP's emergency number straight away, requesting an urgent home visit, or take your baby immediately to the closest accident and emergency department. Once admitted, a chest x-ray and blood tests will be ordered to arrive at a diagnosis.
- Antibiotics are highly effective in managing bacterial pneumonia.
- Viral pneumonia does not respond to antibiotics so the doctors would treat the baby's symptoms. They might prescribe steroids and/or nebulizers to keep the bronchial passages free and to lessen the lung inflammation.
- Bacterial pneumonia can be much more serious, and even fatal, if left untreated.

reflux

Description: Excessive possetting (regurgitating) after feeds; restlessness or pain during feeds.

Explanation: This occurs when the stomach contents, mixed with acid, travel back up the oesophagus, either part way (causing heartburn) or all the way (causing possetting and vomiting). It is partly due to the immature oesophageal sphincter (physiological spincter), and the symptoms naturally lessen as the baby grows older and begins to spend more time upright.

Course of action:

- Try to feed your baby in as upright a position as possible.
- Be sure to wind the baby effectively but gently, and in an upright position.
- Try propping up the head end of the cot as much as you can, without the baby slipping down or sideways.
- Feed little and often to prevent over-feeding and possetting.
- Breastfeeding note: If the mother thinks her baby's spitting up may be related to getting too much milk at feeding, limiting nursing to one breast per feed may help. Another reason for reflux in the breastfed baby is that she may be getting too much milk too quickly.

If the baby gulps or chokes when the mother's let-down occurs, take the baby off the breast for a minute or two; catch the excess milk in a towel, and put the baby back on the breast after the initial flow of milk has passed.

- Formula-fed babies: Offer sips of cool, boiled water throughout the day to temper heartburn. Reflux can sometimes be a sign of food allergy or intolerance, so try switching your brand of formula, if applicable.
- Reflexology can help to ameliorate symptoms and calm down the baby. A practitioner would work down along the oesophageal reflex areas with the intention of lengthening the oesophagus, together with performing a light reflexology workout along the whole gut area.

---

creative healing for reflux

Use a few drops of virgin olive oil. With the fingertips of both hands, stroke the breastbone very lightly in a continuous downwards motion. The fingertips of one hand should follow the fingertips of your other hand. Work straight down from the midpoint of the breastbone to a point midway between the end of the sternum and the belly button. Do this for about four minutes.

---

homeopathy for reflux

Aethusa 30 Indicated if the baby is intolerant of milk. Baby is vomiting or possetting milk as soon as it is swallowed, or in large curds followed by prostration. Worse at 3am to 4am and during the evening, hot weather and dentition. If indicated, try one daily for five days.

The child's constitutional remedy may help, prescribed by a homeopath.

rubella

Description: A pink rash of flat spots spreading across the face and ears, down to the trunk. Accompanied with fever, joint pain and swollen lymph glands in the neck, groin and armpit area.

Explanation: Rubella is airborne and contagious for one week before symptoms appear, until a few days afterwards. It is very rare as most adults have been immunized against it, but it poses a serious risk to pregnant women, especially in the first three months of her gestation, as it can affect the development of certain organs of her unborn child, particularly the hearing apparatus.

Course of action:

- See your doctor. A blood test can confirm the infection.
- Infant paracetamol is prescribed by the doctor to reduce fever, and ibuprofen is given to reduce swelling and redness.
- Keep your child away from playgroups and pregnant women.

---

homeopathy for rubella

Aconite 30 Useful on the first day. Sudden onset. Fever, flushed face, restlessness.

Belladonna 30 Symptoms similar to aconite but after the first day. Fever worse at night. Dilated pupils.

Ferrum Phos 30 Symptoms appear gradually. Fever, rosy spots in the cheeks. Chilly, sweats, wants head kept cool.

Pulsatilla 30 Better for open air. Weepy, desire for company and sympathy. Thirstless. Worse for heat.

slapped cheek (parvovirus B19)

Description: A distinctive pinkish flat rash on the face and trunk (similar to the rubella rash) accompanied with pale lips; occasionally joint pain.

Explanation: Caused by a virus within the red blood cells. There is a two-week incubation period before symptoms appear and they usually disappear within a few weeks, with no lasting effects.

Course of action:
- Infant paracetamol will help reduce joint pain (also give Arnica 30 three times a day for five days).
- Keep the child from rubbing or scratching the rash.
- Homeopathic remedies – similar to the indications for rubella.

teething

Description: Red cheek or cheeks; nappy rash; fever; swollen gums; dribbling; crying and general irritability; discomfort when sucking; disturbed sleep.

Explanation: Babies are not born with their teeth, only teeth buds which sit in the gums and gradually grow out from twelve weeks until the child is three years old. However, there is a huge range of experiences – some children get a tooth as early as eight weeks whilst other mothers visit the dentist at one year to ask for an x-ray to see if the teeth buds are actually there! Teething can happen in clusters – three come along at once – or one by one. Often, the child exhibits all the signs of teething but it can be days, even weeks, before the tooth emerges. Molars are the most painful, but also the last to appear. Children keep their milk teeth until they are about six years old.

Course of action:
- Infant paracetamol ia excellent at reducing the pain and fever that accompanies teething. Along with homeopathy.

- A wooden rattle or board is excellent for little gums to bite down on.
- Equally, a gel teether kept in the fridge can provide relief.
- Some people swear by freezing portions of banana for the baby to bite down on, or you could keep cold carrot sticks ready.
- Nelsons Teetha is a sachet of homeopathic granules which can help, especially with the first, smaller teeth.
- Bonjela is a good ointment which rubs on the gums and provides a mild local anaesthetic effect.
- Teething pendant from India – this has been tried and tested by almost all of my mothers and is wonderfully successful (see page 166).

---

homeopathy for teething

Chamomilla 30 For irritable, wailing, restless babies who are better for being carried. They may be capricious, where nothing seems to suit them. The baby cries when the pain is unbearable. One cheek may be hot and red. Teething may be accompanied with diarrhoea (green stools) and a cough.

Pulsatilla 30 For very weepy, whiny and clingy babies who desire company and to be held. Worse for warm drinks and lying with the head low. Better for cold drink held in the mouth, cold air, walking in the open air and pressure.

Mercurius 30 When there is profuse salivation and foul breath. Profuse sweating at night. Lots of things tend to aggravate and nothing ameliorates the pain of teething.

---

thrush (candidiasis)

Description: Itchiness; white spots (which look like milk curds) in the mouth and on the tongue that cannot be rubbed away; occasionally mouth ulcers; reluctance to feed; could be accompanied by a persistent nappy rash.

Explanation: Thrush occurs when there is an overgrowth of candida bacteria in our intestines and it transforms from a commensal (a natural inhabitant of our gut and skin) to an aggressive fungus. This overgrowth happens when our gut pH balance is disturbed, when our immune system is low or when we kill off the friendly bacteria in our gut with antibiotics (which change the ratio of good and bad bacteria). Oral thrush is the most common form of candidiasis in babies. Candida is a commensal on the surface of the mother's skin, and the baby can pick it up from the mother's breast. Within the baby's mouth is a rich medium of breast milk along with an alkaline pH which makes the thrush proliferate. In this instance, the baby will pass it back to the mother's breast, reinfecting her and making breastfeeding painful (see 'Thrush' in the mother's health section).

Course of action:

- Your GP will probably prescribe an anti-fungal ointment to apply to the baby's mouth, as well as an anti-fungal cream for the mother.
- Offer lots of sips of cool, boiled water throughout the day to keep the mouth washed clean.

---

homeopathy for thrush

There are a few remedies for oral thrush, but one of the most frequently prescribed is:

Kali Mur 30 If the tongue looks mapped or grey or white at the base. There could also be milky white, sticky, thick, slimy or lumpy discharges.

whooping cough (pertussis)

Description: A persistent cough which occurs in episodic runs lasting several minutes and is characterized by a distinctive 'whoop' noise upon inhaling.

Explanation: Often following on the heels of a cold, this is a bacterial infection which irritates the airways and causes an overproduction of mucus, leading to excessive coughing. If coughing is very severe, take your baby to the closest accident and emergency department. Sometimes known as the 100-day cough, it can take several months before finally clearing, and can even return (although without being infectious) if the baby contracts another cold within a year.

homeopathy for whooping cough

Drosera 30c This is one of the principal remedies. One single dose of 30c potency is recommended. There may be a violent, spasmodic cough sounding like a hollow deep barking or a whooping cough. Usually worse after midnight and/or ending in gagging and/or vomiting.

Other useful remedies are:

Ipec 30 Cough with nausea, relieved by vomiting.

Kali Bich 30 Vomiting of yellow, tough and stringy mucus.

Coccus Cacti 30 Vomiting of clear, ropy mucus. Paroxysm of coughing can be warded off with a drink of cold water.

Antimonium Tart 30 Rattling of mucus. Tongue coated thick white; face covered with cold sweat.

See the 'Cough' section for more remedies.

Course of action:

- Steam inhalations can help dislodge mucus and clear the airways, reducing coughing.
- Offer some water during an attack to try to stem the coughing.
- Put your child to sleep in a room with an electric humidifier to keep the air moist.
- See your GP who may prescribe antibiotics.

mother – common postnatal conditions

anaemia

Description: Pale complexion; fatigue and breathlessness; dizzy spells.

Explanation: Anaemia occurs when there is a decrease in the amount of haemoglobin (found in the red blood cells) in your bloodstream, usually arising from dietary deficiencies and bleeding at the birth, although very heavy periods and becoming pregnant soon after a birth can also contribute. Pregnancy is another major reason for anaemia, as the haemoglobin level increases with the blood circulation, but is diluted down by the extra water that is also part of pregnancy. Most people think anaemia means an iron deficiency but it can also relate to low levels of vitamins B_{12} and B_6, selenium, zinc and folic acid.

Course of action:

- Eat a diet rich in iron and minerals. Organic red meat, leafy green vegetables (such as spinach and broccoli), seaweed, pulses and lentils, and dried fruits such as apricots are all ideal.
- Iron supplements may be necessary as well. Floradex is a gentle form which can boost iron levels. (Iron tablets can cause constipation so keep your diet balanced.)
- Mild postnatal anaemia usually disappears naturally as the blood levels normalize and the excess water is shed in the first few weeks after the birth.

- If you bleed heavily during the birth, you may be offered a transfusion or intravenous iron infusions, or you can take a chelated iron preparation.

---

homeopathy: for anaemia

Ferrum Phos 12x If the face is alternately pale or red. This remedy is not clearly indicated but is often useful in acute anaemia.

Ferrum Met 12x When the lips are pale and there is a well-defined cause of blood loss, such as in childbirth. The face may be pale and flush easily.

Calc Phos 12x May be useful after childbirth when regaining strength is proving difficult.

China 12x Following the loss of body fluids, such as blood loss at birth; profuse perspiration.

Phos Acid 12x Following loss of body fluids (prolonged postnatal bleeding) or with an acute illness or associated with emotional trauma. A desire for refreshing food such as fruit and vegetables (to replace the fluid), but may not be thirsty and often tired after eating. Worse for cold and better for sleep.

---

baby blues

Description: Feeling weepy, hopeless, desperate and clingy for no apparent reason, three or four days after the birth.

Explanation: In the post-partum phase, your body is being rocked by massive hormonal changes. As the placental bed leaves the body (through the lochia), levels of the placental hormones, progesterone and oestrogen, return to normal. Given that your oestrogen levels were 300 times higher than normal, this can feel like crashing to rock bottom.

In addition, a new hormone, prolactin (responsible for breast milk), is added to the equation, upsetting the balance yet further.

Course of action:

- Sepia is an effective homeopathic remedy.
- Daily massage with rose otto oil can help. Mix ten drops in a base oil (extra virgin olive or fine almond oil) and gently work along the trunk and limbs for fifteen to twenty minutes; longer if applied by partner.

---

homeopathy for baby blues

Four of the most frequently used remedies for the baby blues are pulsatilla, ignatia, natrun mur and staphisagria. In 30th potency, try repeating three times daily for three days. If the remedy improves things but not enough for recovery, a higher potency may be required; consult a homeopath.

Pulsatilla 30 Indicated if you feel weepy and clingy; if you need a lot of affection, attention and consolation; if you are excessively fearful; if you feel chilly yet find heat intolerable.

Ignatia 30 There may be a feeling of disappointment with silent grief and brooding. Emotions come out in a spasmodic way, with short sobs, sighing and twitching around the mouth with a lot of biting inside the cheek. You might also feel that there is a lump in your throat.

Nat Mur 30 Indicated if there is unexpressed, silent grief; if you feel defensive, closed and cautious; if you feel there is a wall around you. You only want to open up to certain people whom you feel can understand you. You have a tendency to dwell on past disagreeable events. You desire salty foods and you feel worse in the heat of the sun.

Staphisagria 30 If you feel you have suppressed emotions and a sense of indignation about how you have been treated.

---

backache

Description: Throbbing or sharp pain around the upper back and neck, and lower back area.

Explanation: Postnatal back pain is very common, particularly after a long or hard pushing stage, when the shoulder and neck ligaments can become strained. The lumbar (lower back) area is likely to be painful whilst the abdominal muscles are still slack following the pregnancy and unable to support the spine.

Course of action:

- Arnica can help reduce bruised, tense muscles.
- A light shoulder massage from your partner can loosen knots and relieve local tension.
- Direct a showerhead close to the shoulder and neck muscles, and spray with warm water for up to ten minutes.
- Do some gentle stretching to help loosen the muscles and push out any residual lactic acid from the exertions of the birth.
- If your lower back needs support, some support pants which hold in your tummy will give some assistance and relief. Alternatively, try a back support belt. Many pregnancy suppliers sell them for use during and after pregnancy.
- Rest your back by lying on your back with your legs straight up and resting on the wall. This will encourage the lower back to push into the floor and relax.
- Paracetamol will help reduce inflammation and pain. Use sparingly.
- Treatments that can help: osteopathy, cranio-sacral therapy, reflexology, creative healing back treatment, Bowen treatment.

homeopathy for backache

Arnica 30 If you feel bruised and worse with movement.

Kali Carb 30 Indicated for dragging, sore, stitching pain in lower back that feels better for pressure. Also, if you feel worse around 3am, before your period or after long episodes of sitting or walking. This remedy is also indicated if profuse sweating accompanies back pain.

Sepia 30 Indicated if you are worn out, tired or exhausted with an aching, dragging sensation in your lower back. The pain feels better for pressure, worse during the afternoon, at night, before/during menstruation, for bending down and for sitting. You are prone to feeling chilly and irritable, with a desire to be alone.

Antimonium Tart 30 Indicated for violent backache with a dragging feeling; when the slightest movement feels agonizing. You often break out in a cold sweat.

Rhus Tox 30 For a stiff and painful back, where pain is worse on initial movement and better with continued movement.

Bellis Perenis 30 Feels bruised and improves with continued motion. Pain may come on after a long journey sitting in one position.

Bryonia 30 Worse for any movement but better for lying still.

caesarean section scar

Description: Transverse cut along the lower abdominal area (pnannenstiel scar) to allow the baby to be born if a vaginal delivery is not possible.

Course of action:

- After suturing, your diet becomes highly important in protecting the scar. Constipation brings unnecessary and excessive pushing, which places the scar under strain. A stool softener such as Lactulose will be medically indicated but you should follow a low-fibre diet to help keep everything soft. Linseeds, prunes, figs, dates, raisins and compote will help enormously.
- Avoid hot baths, which can cause inflammation, but you can take them between 34 and 36 degrees centigrade with ten drops of tea tree oil (antiseptic) and/or lavender oil (anti-inflammatory).
- Drink lots of water to keep your body and bowel hydrated.
- Go to the toilet as soon as you feel the need to open your bowels. The stools will become drier the longer they remain in the bowel, meaning you'll have to push harder.
- When you do go to the toilet, hold a sanitary pad to your abdominal scar and push as gently as you can.
- Take iron supplements and 500mg of vitamin C daily. There are specific postnatal preparations that can help.
- It's also very important to look after your lung and respiratory health. A chest infection – with its inherent coughing – will place unwanted pressure on the intra-abdominal wall. Steam inhalations with a couple of drops of tea tree and rosemary oil will help cleanse your respiratory system. Note: Do not use tea tree oil if you are taking a homeopathic remedy as strong essential oils like tea tree or rosemary will reduce or cancel out the potency of homeopathic medicines.

constipation

Description: Difficulty, inability or no urge to pass stools after three or more days. Stools are hard, solid and formed.

Explanation: The main culprits are usually dehydration, hormonal imbalance or holding on too long before going to the toilet, causing the stools to dry out and become harder to pass.

Course of action:

- Plenty of water and a high-fibre diet will work wonders. Choose fibrous fruits like pears, apples, melon, figs, prunes, dates and raisins; and vegetables such as celery, squash, broccoli, cabbage, carrots, parsnips or runner beans.
- A mild glycerine suppository can help ease the movement of your bowels.
- The seven-minute creative healing treatment which works on the dimples in the sacrum is also very effective. You could ask your partner to perform it on you daily (see page 93).
- Light exercise – like walking or swimming – can help massage and stimulate the bowel.
- Reflexology – ask the therapist to place emphasis on treating the colon reflex areas.
- Several yoga poses can help regularize the bowel. The Child pose helps open the bowel; the Rock pose can help ease indigestion.
- Digestive enzymes can help boost your digestive health and act as a deterrent to future episodes – try Dr Udo or Biocare.
- Probiotics help maintain gut balance – choose from Solgar or Biocare.

See baby 'Constipation' for more remedies.

homeopathy for constipation

Unless otherwise indicated, the remedy should be taken three times a day until a good response is obtained, then reduced to twice, and finally to once a day as the condition improves.

Aluminium Metallicum 6c If you pass hard, marble-like masses and have to strain very hard, try once a day for three days.

Nux Vom 6c If you have a feeling of incomplete emptying of your bowels, take once a day for three days.

Silicea 6c For a bashful stool - one that recedes when partly expelled - take once a day for three days.

Nux Vomica 30 If you're hooked on laxatives, nux vomica may help break the habit. It's also indicated if you have frequent ineffectual urging, or pass out small quantities of stool at each attempt. You feel as if part remains unexpelled, compelling you to try to pass stool frequently.

Sepia 6c Stools are large and hard, with ineffectual straining. Abdomen feels full.

Opium 6c Indicated if you rarely get an urge to pass a stool, where there seems to be insensitivity and inactivity in the rectum, and the stool recedes after being partly expelled.

Aesculus 6c If you have to pass stool with difficulty because it is large and hard - it feels as if sticks are being passed.

Sulphur 30 If your stools are hard, dark and dry, with burning at the anus.

Nat Mur 30 If you pass a crumbly stool that causes rectal bleeding, smarting and soreness.

Graphites 30 Take this remedy if stools look like round balls stuck together with mucus and are painful to pass. There may be an absence of stool for days, perhaps with associated anal fissures and cracks.

cystitis

Description: Burning or stinging sensation when passing water; lower abdominal pain; increased frequency and urgency of urination; occasionally, blood in the urine.

Explanation: The female urethra is very short and therefore easily vulnerable to infection from the anus, particularly following the bruising and compression of the tissue during childbirth. Postnatal cystitis is very common.

Course of action:

- Make your urine more alkaline by squeezing lemon juice into your drinking water, and/or adding some cranberry juice. Drink little and often – although this means going to the toilet more often (which is initially painful), it will help dilute the urine and so reduce the stinging sensation. It also means you are likely to neutralize and flush out the infection faster. Pass water as soon as you feel the urge – don't 'hold on'.
- Avoid caffeine.
- Creative healing – heat can be taken off the abdomen by using the cooling breeze, abdominal toning, pelvic drainage, the female treatment and a kidney treatment. Whilst a few of these procedures can be done at home, you might find it easier to visit a creative healer, if there is one in your area.
- Reflexology – concentrate on the kidney and bladder reflexes.
- There are plenty of over-the-counter medications such as Cystemme.
- If symptoms persist for three days or there is blood in the urine, see your doctor. If left untreated, the infection can travel up to your kidneys and cause a serious kidney infection.

gentle first year

Cantharis 30c Take twice a day for three days if you have a lot of urgency and frequency, and a burning pain before, during and immediately after urination. Urine could be hot and low in volume. The pains come on suddenly and are violent and spasmodic. The bladder never feels empty in spite of a constant desire to pass water. The pains are often aggravated by cold drinks and you may have a burning thirst.

Staphisagria 30 Take for frequent urination; where there is an ineffectual urge to urinate; urging and pain after urination; a sensation as if a drop of urine were continually rolling along the channel; burning in urethra. Often indicated where there is a feeling of having been abused and where strong feelings were not expressed, or after a mechanical childbirth with pain afterwards and possibly stitches.

deep vein thrombosis

Description: Swelling or pain in the legs, particularly the calf area.

Explanation: Caused by a blood clot that develops in the major veins. It can be life-threatening if a thrombosis fragments and travels to the lungs. The blood's coagulability (ability to clot) increases in pregnancy, leading to the blood thickening and circulation becoming more sluggish. Periods of inactivity – such as a long labour (twenty-four hours or more) – can compound this sluggishness.

Course of action:
- See your GP **immediately** or go to hospital.
- Drink lots of water to keep the blood from thickening.
- Your doctor will prescribe a blood thinner like 75mg aspirin daily.
- If you have had a Caesarean or pre-existing varicose veins, wear support stockings.

- Put ten drops of Cypress essential oil in a small bowl of water and wring out a flannel; then apply cold compresses all the way down the legs. (Important note: always work in a downwards direction, never up towards the heart and lungs as this will prevent any clots being pushed upwards.)
- Do not sit with your legs crossed.
- Use creative healing as first aid: Ask your partner or friend to create and apply a cooling breeze with cupped hands, coated in olive oil, drawing downwards in a kind of stroking movement – the hands should not touch your skin and the palms should face the leg that is being treated. Note: It is difficult to remove heat from yourself: You have to ask for help from a friend or partner.

---

homeopathy for deep vein thrombosis

Arnica 200c Take four-hourly during the day for two to three days until the pain subsides. It is an anti-inflammatory and good for pain relief.

Kali.Mur 6c Take four times a day for seven days, as an alternative option.

Note: Also see a professional homeopath who can prescribe on a deeper level.

---

dropped arches

Description: When the arch of the foot flattens, resulting in a 'waddling' walk.

Explanation: This is a reasonably common side-effect of the increased amounts of progesterone circulating around the body during pregnancy, but if left unchecked can lead the foot to rotate inwards and cause knee pain.

Course of action:

- The foot will naturally tighten up as the level of progesterone drops after birth, but a yoga walk can help speed things along: Standing barefoot, arch your feet like claws, trying to keep the arches as far away from the floor as possible. Walk around the room for five minutes as a time.
- See a podiatrist: They might suggest and design a special insole to support your arches; or better still they might teach you specific exercises and correct your gait.

dyspareunea

Description: When sexual intercourse is painful or uncomfortable following birth.

Explanation: Most often this condition occurs following a vaginal tear or episiotomy, when the scar is new and thick. But even in instances where the birth went smoothly, without tearing or instrumental intervention, there is still bruising and internal stretching. If those bruised pelvic floor muscles are left to heal without intervention, the bruising can cause congestion in the local areas, and the muscles of the vagina can go into contraction, making penetration painful.

Course of action:

- Where scarring is the problem, a fascial unwind will help (see 'Keloids').
- Following bruising, a pelvic drainage massage (see page 65) can clear congestion from the area and allow the muscles to drain and relax. This should be done preventatively four to six weeks after all birth experiences (instrumental or normal).

haemorrhoids (piles)

Description: Engorged veins located in the lowest part of the rectum, just within the anal canal (internal), although they can sometimes protrude (external).

Explanation: Usually a result of increased pressure from the pregnant uterus on the pelvic veins, causing back pressure in the blood flow around the pelvic and rectal area and leading to dilatation and engorgement of the piles. Can also be attributed to constipation and prolonged pushing at the birth.

Course of action:

- There is a specific creative healing haemorrhoid treatment that can be applied externally to the sacrum and coccyx. I like to call it the haemorrhoid lift! It is very efficient at reducing and healing haemorrhoids (see Resources for do-at-home DVD).
- Going on all fours, isolating the anal sphincter muscles and contracting them in three stages with the breath can help prevent piles during pregnancy and cure them afterwards. This is the only pre-natal pelvic floor exercise I recommend.
- Vaginal stretching and oiling will also help reduce pressure on the rectal mucosa.

homeopathy for haemorrhoids

Hamamelis 30c Take twice a day for three to four days. It is good for piles that occur towards the end of pregnancy and during birth, especially if they are associated with bleeding, soreness and bruising.

Sepia 6c For external and internal piles that may be hard and large. The piles may be associated with constipation. There may be a sense of having a lump in the rectum with pains that shoot upward. There could be an almost constant oozing from the rectum with a sensation of bearing down.

Kali Carb 30 Take for piles that are large and protrude when passing stool or coughing. Often caused by childbirth, these are worse for being touched, and the acute pain and inflammation is relieved by hot applications.

Lachesis 30 Throbbing pain in the haemorrhoids, which are hypersensitive and relieved by cold applications. The haemorrhoids may be bluish/purple.

Ignatia 30c Good for internal piles that cause shooting pains that appear after birth.

- Ayurvedic wisdom expounds wearing a sanitary towel soaked in warm olive oil. Lie down on a plastic mat or towel, ensuring that the sanitary pad is in contact with the piles, for an hour a day.
- Cold compresses for twenty minutes, three times a day, can lessen the discomfort.
- A sitz bath can be helpful. Sit in a bath with 15cm of tepid water and twenty drops of cypress essential oil for twenty minutes. In naturopathy, it is common practice to immerse the affected part in water warmer or cooler than body temperature. Traditionally, a sitz bath looks like a shallow bucket, which contains enough water to immerse the essential bits!

- Take a cotton wool make-up remover pad and soak in witch hazel. Tuck it into the crack between the buttocks to reduce the swelling and restore comfort.
- Avoid constipation by drinking lots of water and eating a medium-fibre diet.

incontinence (urinary and bowel)

Description: Inability to control or stop the urge to urinate or open bowels.

Explanation: An incredibly common complaint and more likely with second and subsequent pregnancies, where the mother's pelvic floor has already been stretched. It's also more likely with a large baby (9lb or more) or if you were pushing for more than an hour in labour because the chronic pressure causes damage to the bladder neck and/or some of the muscles in the rectal sphincter.

Course of action:
- Pelvic floor exercises are best, but very difficult for the first six weeks, as bruising and overstretching can make it hard to feel anything. I advise a Pilates-based modification on the traditional exercises. Lie on your back with your knees bent and hips raised, but instead of concentrating on contracting and releasing the three distinct pelvic floor areas (urethra, vagina, rectum), instead focus on squeezing the lower abdominals. These are much bigger muscle masses, which you can more easily feel working, and because everything is connected by fascia, they will automatically pull on and contract the pelvic floor for you. In the first six weeks, this is by far the better option as it stops mothers from panicking that they can't feel these tiny movements. Move on to more specific pelvic floor exercises after six weeks (see page 146).
- If the incontinence is severe or not responding to a standard pelvic floor routine, it is possible to use weights prescribed by a physiotherapist.

These are inserted into the vagina and you walk around with them in, starting with ten minutes and building up to an hour or so. The idea is that the muscles in and surrounding the vagina are forced to exercise and contract in order to retain the weights.

- You might also like to try the Epino, which is popular in Europe, particularly France, and Israel. The balloon is inflated and inserted into the vagina. You then have to squeeze the vaginal muscles to pop the Epino back out. For more information visit www.epino.com.
- There are specialist incontinence nurses who can be consulted.

---

homeopathy for incontinence

Arsenicum Album 30 Indicated if you are anxious and restless; chilly; thirsty for large quantities or frequent small quantities of fluids. You feel better for hot drinks, warmth of bed and lying down; worse for change of temperature, cold, damp and exertion after midnight, especially if woken up at 3am. Also worse on laughing or walking. Incontinence can be brought on by becoming chilled.

Nat Mur 30 Symptoms are worse for laughing, coughing, sneezing, walking and exertion.

Pulsatilla 30 Symptoms are worse for coughing, laughing, sneezing and walking. You may be weepy, clingy and whiney with a desire for open air. Condition is aggravated by heat.

Sepia 30 Symptoms are worse for coughing, laughing, sneezing and walking. You feel chilly; prefer to be alone; angry. You may crave vinegar. Condition may be worse around the time of the menstrual period.

Causticum 30 Symptoms are worse for coughing and sneezing, and may come on after becoming chilled.

---

insomnia

Description: Inability to fall asleep, despite tiredness; waking at the slightest sound.

Explanation: It's quite common for new mothers to find it hard to sleep in the early weeks. The expectation of getting up to do the next feed can make it hard to relax into sleep, and even when sleep does come, it can be easily disturbed by a snuffle that you hear down the baby monitor! This can be attributed to anxiety and wildly changing hormone levels.

Course of action:

- Sleep in the day when the baby does. For the first few weeks, it's important to adjust to a series of catnaps as the baby will be regularly feeding every few hours, even through the night.

- When the baby is three or more weeks old some mothers like to introduce a bottle of formula or express some milk to allow their partner to do a night feed. This allows you to miss a feed and enjoy one longer spell of sleep before having to do the next one. On the other hand, remember that it is normal for babies to wake up during the night and that, due to the hormones released during breastfeeding, you may sleep better and deeper after you have breastfed. Also, your breasts can become engorged and uncomfortable if you go for five to six hours without feeding, so weigh up the pros and cons.

- Put some lavender essential oil into a burner and let it burn for several hours in your room before going to bed.

- Try listening to my sleep tape with visualizations that I originally recorded for one of my mothers. Many of my pregnant mothers claim to find it impossible to stay awake during my tape as they find my voice so relaxing!

- Ask your partner to give you a luxurious body massage every few nights or so, which will lead to sleep.

- If the baby has trouble settling, which upsets you, ask your partner to settle the baby after a couple of feeds, and put in some earplugs.

- Alternatively, if you are formula-feeding, ask a family member or professional nanny agency – such as Night Nannies – to come in and cover a night shift for you for one or more nights a week, moving up to once a fortnight as the baby begins to sleep for longer spells.

---

homeopathy for insomnia

A remedy may need to be prescribed based on the cause of the insomnia and/or any clear emotional symptoms. However, if the insomnia has come on mainly because the habit of sleep has been lost after many sleepless nights nursing the baby then cocculus indicus may be useful. When cocculus indicus is indicated there are symptoms of trembling with tiredness and a feeling of being much worse from fresh air and physical exertion. There is a general numb feeling, as if specific parts have gone to sleep.

---

keloids

Description: Thick, raised, 'rope' scar – following Caesarean, episiotomy or vaginal tear. Keloids can occur on any area of the body that has sustained a surgical or accidental cut. Some individuals have an increased keloid tendency. It has been noted that Asian and African races have a greater tendency to exhibit skin keloid formation because they have a higher collagen content in their skin.

Explanation: It is not unusual for scarring to adhere to the immediate fat and muscle fascias beneath the skin. Your obstetrician will have taken every care to stitch each layer separately so that the skin, muscle and fat levels sit separately on top of each other, like rolling balloons. Scarring is genetically determined, however, and some people heal better than others. If scarring is pronounced and adheres to separate fascias, it can act like a cascade – with the fascia of the abdominal muscle, the rectus abdominus, tethering to the peritoneal fascia beneath, which in turn pulls on the uterus, cervix and ultimately ovaries. Some people find that where the skin fascia adheres to the muscle sheath of the rectus abdominus, it can eventually pull on the front of the neck and at the base of the skull. This eventual attachment might give rise to neurological problems.

Course of action: A fascial unwinding (a gentle lifting and rolling of the fascia) can be performed from six weeks to thin and loosen the scar. Usually only one session is needed but occasionally a follow-up is helpful.

loss of/low libido

Description: No desire for sexual contact, from kisses and cuddles to intercourse.

Explanation: This is one of the most common and yet least discussed aspects of the immediate post-partum phase. Libido can be one of the casualties of the hormonal drop that follows birth, as oestrogen and progesterone levels decline dramatically. Also, from a practical standpoint, sexual intercourse is ill-advised before three weeks after the birth as the vaginal area is often still very bruised, tender and stretched (even without tearing or an episiotomy), the lochia (bleeding) is strong and there is a higher risk of infection. Many doctors say sex is fine any time after the six-week postnatal check, when the birth passages and the skin of the perineum have healed.

Course of action:

- Make sure you have accepted the birth experience and forgiven any intervention which was traumatic to go through. I strongly recommend moving through the birth acceptance visualization (page 52) before you resume sexual relations.
- Remember, your partner may have conflicting emotions about the birth too, if it was very painful, long or there was an emergency.

Fathers experience birth vividly as witnesses, so allow your partner to discuss his feelings – which may range from anger to powerlessness.

- Your body is still recovering up to twelve weeks after the birth, so take your time to rediscover each other. Giving and receiving sensual massage is an excellent way to welcome each other back into a sexual relationship even – or especially – if it does not lead to intercourse in the early weeks. Using essential oils such as ylang ylang, jasmine, neroli, sandalwood and patchouli, either on their own or in a sensitive blend, will help with arousal.
- I recommend the Ayurvedic herb Ashwagandha (*Withania somnifera*) to both mothers and fathers to really give libido a boost.
- Once the baby is a few months old and the breastfeeding schedule is not quite so intense, try to go out with your partner for a night. Even just going two miles down the road and having an intimate dinner will give you some breathing space from 'just' being parents, and allow you some crucial time together as a couple.
- If you are breastfeeding and nurturing another life, it can be difficult to then shift into a sexual role. If you still suffer from low libido or feel very conflicted about yourself as a sexual person (which is common in the year after birth), you might like to see a relationship counsellor who can talk through your fears and anxieties.

---

homeopathy for loss of/low libido

Loss of libido may be the result of one or a number of issues, such as physical trauma, exhaustion, hormonal imbalance or more complex emotional issues. Sepia is a frequently indicated remedy when there is indifference to loved ones; irritability associated with a preference to be alone; exhaustion yet feels better for vigorous exercise. There may be a feeling of chilliness and of something heavy inside that is dragging you down.

---

mother & baby health a-z

mastitis

Description: Inflammation and redness of the breast tissue, leading to localized, shooting pain during and between feeds; tender lumps in the breast; fever and flu-symptoms.

Explanation: Mastitis occurs due to blocked milk ducts (when a milk duct is not fully cleared during a feed and the residual milk becomes compacted and hard, leading to tender lumps). If the milk duct is not drained, the milk begins to seep through the lining of the milk duct into the surrounding breast tissue causing inflammation, fever, aches and pains and other flu-like symptoms.

Course of action:

- The most important thing is to continue to feed. Regular feeding will help drain and clear the milk.
- Check your baby's latch – incorrect positioning can lead to the baby not feeding properly or fully, leaving milk at the end of each feed.
- Check you are not taking the baby off the breast too quickly. Allow the baby to stay on as long as she needs to.
- Always offer both sides at each feed and begin the feed on the side you last finished on to ensure complete drainage of each breast.
- Breastfeed the baby frequently on the affected side, every two hours if possible, including at night.
- Varying the nursing positions, e.g. football hold, side-lying, may help to relieve a plugged duct.
- The baby is the best unplugger of milk ducts, but if the feed still has not drained the affected milk duct, using a breast pump may help.
- Drink lots of fluids.
- Paracetamol, aspirin and ibuprofen will reduce temperature and inflammation.
- Gently massage the outer perimeters of the breast tissue (avoiding the nipple area) in a clockwise motion, working towards the armpit (this is where the breast lymphatics drain). Perform this massage for five

minutes, using a good-quality base oil such as extra virgin olive oil or fine almond oil.

- Placing warm, wet flannels on the breast before a feed can help loosen and dislodge the milk. Alternatively, direct warm water from a shower head at close range to the breast for ten to fifteen minutes.
- Make sure you are wearing a well-fitting, supportive breastfeeding bra, and do not wear an underwired bra as this can compress the milk ducts.
- Antibiotics may be necessary if the mastitis does not respond to the above within a couple of days (they are safe for the baby, as they are excreted in breastmilk in extremely minute quantities).

homeopathy for mastitis

In the early stages of inflammation try bryonia or belladonna.

Bryonia 30 If there is pain that is worse on movement (you must support the breast with a good soft bra). The pains may feel like a stitch or a tear.

Belladonna 30 Indicated if the breast is bright red, hot and tender. There is a rapid onset, with burning, throbbing pains made worse with sudden, jarring movements, and the breast is very sensitive to the lightest touch. Part of the breast may be affected with red streaks.

Phytolacca 30 When the breast has become hard like a stone. There are painful, very hard lumps that may be associated with a past injury. An abscess could be forming.

Hepar Sulphuris 30 Indicated if there has been suppuration (the formation of pus). There will be a feeling of intense heat and throbbing in the breast.

Description: Bright pink or raw-looking nipples. There could be dark ecchymosis (evidence of subcutaneous bleeding) around the areola.

Explanation: In almost every case, sore nipples can be attributed to a poor latch, although in some instances, it is due to thrush (see 'Thrush', pages 270 and 303).

Course of action:

- See a midwife or breastfeeding specialist to really study your baby's position and latching technique. Often, the difference is just a matter of centimetres but the change can be huge. Once this is right the problem should resolve itself.
- Express some milk (manually) before feeding to stimulate the let-down reflex before putting the baby to the breast. Or, if only one nipple is sore, begin to nurse on the other side until let-down occurs, then switch the baby to the affected side (ensure good position and latch).
- Express and rub some of your milk onto the nipples and allow them to air dry after every feed.
- Some mothers like to use a lanolin-based barrier cream such as Lansinoh or Kamillosan (available from pharmacies and supermarkets). (Do wash it off before the next feed, but I would advise you to, as the commercial varieties do contain some preservatives.)
- If the pain becomes too much, don't give up. Express your milk and feed the baby with this for a short time.
- Avoid nipple shields as they prevent the baby from getting a good mouthful of breast and therefore from breastfeeding properly, and can cause other breastfeeding problems.
- If the nipples are still sore, ask your midwife or health visitor to check you haven't got thrush. If you have taken antibiotics, the thrush may be systemic (in your bloodstream) rather than local (sitting on top of the breast).

over-scarring

Description: When scarring exceeds the original suture line and impacts upon surrounding areas or adheres to underlying tissues – usually following a vaginal tear or episiotomy.
Explanation: For some people, the scar tissue continues to grow beyond where it is required. This can be compounded if the obstetrician has not left a small margin for any extra tissue growth. Genetics also play a role in this condition.

Course of action:

- A fascial unwind is the first response (see page 291), but stretching exercises can also make a dramatic difference. Use the vaginal oils recommended on the antenatal gentle birth method programme to lubricate the vagina. Starting with two fingers, gently press ten times against each of the side and back walls. As you progress, move up to deeper finger insertion and more repetitions.

- An Epino (see page 287) will do the same thing – gently inflate the balloon inside the vagina but remember it does not have the same intelligence as the manual method. Most people have an imbalance in their gait, which means one side of muscle wall is correspondingly thicker and more rigid than the other. The Epino cannot register this difference – only how much the balloon's surface area can expand – so it simply continues to expand the vaginal space by inflating into the stretched side without breaking down the density in the resistant side.

- In severe cases, surgery may be required.

persistent bleeding

Description: Bleeding that continues beyond the normal range for lochia (six weeks plus).

Explanation: Your doctor will do a clinical examination, looking for tenderness in the lower abdominal area. Even if this feels okay, they will probably still do a vaginal examination to check for tenderness and to see if the cervix is painful. Even if the lower vagina feels fine, there can often be painful pelvic inflammation higher up. This is due to bruising from the birth and is common. If left untreated, an infection can develop in these bruised tissues. At other times, the inflammation is due to an infection – usually E. Coli from the gut or bacterioides. These usually inhabit the gut, but when tissues become devitalized (bruised), they can migrate out of the thin, inflamed gut wall and land in the 'pouch of Douglas', which is the area of peritonium right behind the uterus.

Course of action: Antibiotics. Some homeopaths will argue they can treat the condition but I prefer not to take any chances as there is always the threat of the infection developing into puerperal sepsis (septicaemia).

---

homeopathy for persistent bleeding

Consult a homeopath. Homeopathic remedies can be really useful alongside conventional medicine.

---

postnatal depression

Description: Feeling hopeless, anxious, unable to cope or overwhelmed by motherhood and the baby; fatigue; weepy and clingy; resentful; feeling detached and not bonded to the baby; mania; loss of libido.

Explanation: The levels of progesterone and oestrogen which were buoyed up during pregnancy (up to 300 times for oestrogen) drop dramatically in the first few days after birth as the placenta is expelled. Then there is a significant increase in prolactin, the hormone responsible for bringing in the milk. The huge shifts take a toll on the mother's emotions and can induce the very common baby blues (see page 40). Postnatal depression differs from this in that it lasts for much longer and can be difficult to recognize as it manifests itself in ways other than classic weepiness.

Course of action:

- Make sure you have accepted the birth experience and forgiven any intervention which was traumatic to go through. I strongly recommend moving through the birth acceptance visualization in the first few weeks after birth (see page 52).

- I strongly advise a massage with mood-elevating essential oils like rose otto (ten drops) plus rosemary (five drops) administered by either your partner or a therapist every day for at least fifteen minutes for the first few weeks. Touch is a potent healing force and will make you feel cared for, and the endorphins released will help lift your mood. It is also a precious opportunity in which to focus on how you feel and on healing your body. A massage would give you a much needed break from your new non-stop role as mother.
- Please relax the pressure on yourself to get life 'back to normal' as soon as possible. Of course, it is more difficult if you already have another child and want to minimize disruption to them, but racing around and avoiding your anxieties or fears will not make them go away. Often, doctors are more concerned about the mother who insists everything is absolutely fine and presents a perfect face to the world than the weepy mother who says she cannot cope.
- In extreme instances, postnatal depression goes a step further and becomes puerperal psychosis. This is characterized by mania and rapid, broken speech. It affects roughly one in every 500 women, and is treated with medication and, usually, hospitalization.

homeopathy for postnatal depression

Homeopathy can be highly effective when treating this condition and there are many useful remedies, so if home prescribing does not help, contact a homeopath for assistance. (See 'Baby Blues', page 40 for more remedies.)

Sepia 30 Indifference to loved ones, angry, sarcastic, impatient with a desire to be alone.

Kali Carb 30 Argues with family and has a fear of losing control. Dogmatic with a strong sense of duty. Emotions are felt in the stomach like a blow.

scoliosis

Description: When the spine takes on a sideways bend either to the right or the left. This is often described as an S-shaped spine. There are varying degrees of scoliosis. Some are not easily noticed while others reduce the height of the individual.

Explanation: A baby can be born with congenital scoliosis or it can be acquired in childhood or adulthood by bad posture; nutritional deficiencies that lead to weak spinal ligaments; or minor degrees of intervertebral disc displacement or hypertrophied muscles on one side of the spine that pull the spine out of alignment.

Course of action:

- Investigative x-rays or MRI scans can rule out any serious underlying causes.
- Exercise: Corrective yoga or Pilates.
- Creative healing: The treatment of repositioning substance between the vertebrae is one of the four principles of creative healing. With this treatment I have been able to correct varying degrees of scoliosis and restore the contours of the spine into a straight line going down the midline of the back. I would love to share a case history of one of my pregnant mothers whom I remember with fondness.

Treating Scoliosis through Creative Healing

My patient had quite a marked scoliosis that had been diagnosed since childhood. I took on the challenge and enrolled my team members Debbie and Marion to treat her once or twice a week, slowly remoulding the substance between the vertebrae of her back. She received treatments throughout her pregnancy. Needless to say, she had a wonderful birth and we continued her treatments for three months afterwards. One of the best moments was when she arrived to see me in a strappy dress. When I complimented her on how wonderful she looked, she said that she had never been able to wear this kind of dress before. I was truly chuffed!

She later told me that in her teens, an orthopaedic surgeon had wanted to operate and insert rods in her back to straighten the spine but she had declined the operation. She was so pleased with creative healing that she was keen to set up a meeting with that very same orthopaedic surgeon so that I could discuss and demonstrate how creative healing had corrected her scoliosis.

Since then, whenever I assess mothers who arrive at the clinic for birth preparation, I look for all degrees of scoliosis and treat them! This highlights the most important part of the the 'Jeyarani Way' gentle birth method of birth preparation – and that is to treat the whole person.

stretchmarks

Description: Vivid red, light-brown or dark-brown striations across the tummy, hips and upper thighs.

Explanation: Stretchmarks occur when the skin is stretched past its natural elasticity – most commonly during rapid weight gain or weight loss or in normal individuals during pregnancy. The marks fade to pale silver over time and are not itchy. It's not unusual for stretchmarks to become apparent after pregnancy, as the skin shrinks back to pre-pregnant size. Stretchmarks are now understood to be genetically determined, so if your mother has them, it's likely you will be prone to them.

Course of action:

- Controlling your weight – particularly during pregnancy – will help.
- Make sure to moisturize and nourish the skin after the birth to keep it supple whilst it reverts to its pre-pregnant shape.
- Midwives around the world extol the rich virtues of cocoa butter.
- I advocate Ayurvedic oils which deeply nourishes the skin both before and after pregnancy.
- Eat a diet rich in calcium and essential fats like the omega-3 oils to boost the skin's natural elasticity.
- After your six-week check, begin a gentle exercise routine to improve your muscle tone and give your skin a lift.

---

homeopathy for stretchmarks

Calc Fluor 6c is useful to take during pregnancy as it assists skin elasticity. It can be used as part of the pregnancy tissue salt programme.

Description: A full tear of the vaginal wall, going all the way through to the rectum.

Explanation: It will be immediately apparent to the obstetrician and midwife at the birth if you have had a third-degree tear. You will probably be taken into theatre for suturing by a senior obstetrician.

Course of action:

- Once the tear has been stitched, diet becomes highly important in protecting the area from constipation and excessive pushing. A stool softener such as Lactulose will be medically indicated but you should follow a low residue diet to help keep everything soft. Linseeds, prunes, figs, dates, raisins and compote will help enormously.
- Avoid hot baths, which can cause inflammation, but you can take them at 35 degrees centigrade with ten to fifteen drops of tea tree oil (antiseptic) and/or lavender (anti-inflammatory).
- Drink lots of water to keep the body – and bowel – hydrated.
- Go to the toilet as soon as you feel the need to open the bowels. The stools will become harder to expel the longer they remain in the rectum. It is not good to strain at opening your bowels when a third-degree tear is beginning to heal. You will also find it helpful to hold a sanitary pad to support your perineum and push as gently as you can.
- Take 500mg of vitamin C daily.
- It's also very important to look after your lung and respiratory health. A chest infection – with its inherent coughing – will place unwanted pressure on the pelvic floor when the tissues are in the healing phase. Steam inhalations with a couple of drops of tea tree oil will help cleanse your respiratory system. Note: Do not use tea tree oil if you are taking a homeopathic remedy as strong oils reduce or cancel their potency.

thrush (candidiasis)

Description: White spots on and around the nipples; red inflamed breast tissue; burning or a 'cut glass' pain when feeding; often accompanied or preceded by vaginal thrush – including itchiness, a thick white discharge and strong odour.

Explanation: Thrush occurs when the body's alkaline balance is disturbed and becomes more acidic (often following illness, antibiotics or during the hormonal changes of pregnancy), allowing the candida fungus to flourish and spread.

Course of action:

- If you have thrush of the breast tissue and are breastfeeding, go to your GP to check that your baby is not also infected, as you may be reinfecting each other. If you both have it, you will be prescribed a topical anti-fungal cream, and some drops for the baby.
- If you have vaginal thrush you can buy over-the-counter creams such as Canesten.
- If vaginal thrush persists beyond three to four weeks, see your GP. If it is confirmed as thrush, your GP can give you a stronger prescription or some pessaries.
- Avoid tampons whilst you have vaginal thrush, and use condoms during sexual intercourse to prevent infecting your partner.
- Always wipe from front to back when you go to the toilet.
- Follow a low-carbohydrate, low-sugar diet to keep sugar levels low,

and avoid fizzy drinks. Eat plenty of steamed green vegetables and drink a glass of juiced greens a day as these will alkalinize your gut.

- Probiotics like acidophilus capsules from Biocare, taken daily, will help control and regulate your 'friendly' bacteria levels and keep a check on the growth of the fungus candida (which occurs naturally in our bodies).
- Live yoghurts and probiotic drinks are also easy to get hold of, but have quite high sugar levels. Try Kephir, a version of probiotics that you can make at home. (Read more at the website: www.thekephirshop.co.uk)
- Midwives recommend placing a couple of spoonfuls of live yoghurt into the vagina before going to bed at night (make sure your lochia has stopped and, where applicable, your episiotomy scar has healed before you do this).
- A couple of drops of tea tree oil in your bath water will help. Make sure the water temperature is not too warm as this will encourage the candida to thrive.

---

homeopathy for thrush

Kali Mur 6x If the discharge is milky white, thick and profuse.
Pulsatilla 6x If the discharge is creamy, thick and burning.
Sepia 6x If there is a lumpy, milky discharge. There can be dryness of the vagina and an aversion to sex.
Sulphur 30 The vagina may be itchy, red and sore with a burning pain. Symptoms may be made worse with bathing and heat.

vaginal prolapse

Description: The first and second degrees of vaginal prolapse are hidden from sight; this is when the cervix drops a little way into the high vaginal area. In extreme cases, the entire cervix is seen prolapsed outside the vagina. This is rarely seen in the UK nowadays, due to early intervention by gynaecologists who would surgically correct the vaginal prolapse. In post-menopausal women, vaginal prolapse can occur due to poor pelvic muscle tone, usually caused by poor nutrition and lack of physical activity. Some women refuse operative intervention and resort to using a vaginal pessary (a rubber or plastic ring) to keep the cervix and uterus in place.

Explanation: This could happen to varying degrees after each and every birth, until the pelvic area has recovered from bruising and the uterus has contracted back to its normal size.

Course of action: The creative healing pelvic lift can remedy the situation, at two, four and six weeks after the birth (see page 65).

---

homeopathy for vaginal prolapse

Remedies used straight after the birth to assist recovery may help reduce the occurrence of a vaginal prolapse. Trauma remedies such as arnica 12x may assist recovery once a prolapse has occurred, and constitutional remedies may help recovery.

---

varicose veins

Description: Enlargement of the veins, most often found in the legs (behind the knee) and the vulva.

Explanation: Inefficient venous return to the heart (often due to the weight of the pregnant uterus on the veins) contributes to back pressure on the veins, causing swelling and engorgement.

Course of action:

- Wear support stockings.
- Drink lots of water – at least two litres a day.
- Do not sit with your legs crossed and do not stand for long periods.
- Rest with your legs above your heart level for at least fifteen minutes a day.
- Lie on the floor with your bottom against the wall and your legs stretched straight above you, resting on the wall. Rest your head and shoulders on a cushion.
- Help reduce inflammation by massaging the legs in a downward direction only. Use an essential oil mix of ten drops of cypress and ten drops of lavender blended with 30ml of virgin olive oil. I would recommend the creative healing massage technique as outlined below.

creative healing massage

Using both hands, lightly massage the legs in a downward direction only to gently drain the legs. Hands should be open and cupped. Start from mid-thigh and move down to the ankles. Repeat for five minutes on each leg. Very gently massage downwards with your fingertips in the deep space behind the knees (this is called the popliteal fossa and contains a specific drainage filter area for the lower limb).

homeopathy for varicose veins

There are many homeopathic remedies for varicose veins. Repeat the chosen remedy three times daily for a week. If the veins feel improved, continue taking the remedy once a day for a further two to three weeks.

Calc Carb 12x For vulval varicosities. Better for heat and for lying down. Worse for cold, damp, draughts, exertion, fresh air and tight clothes.

Calc Fluor 12x If the veins are aggravated by cold, damp weather, and if the tissues around them have become worn out, flabby and lax.

Carbo Veg 12x For varicose veins of the leg, thigh and/or vulva that feel better in cool, fresh air and worse on exertion and in humidity.

Ferrum Met 12x For swollen, painful varicose veins of the leg, thigh and/or foot. Often accompanied by anaemia and tiredness.

Hamamelis 12x For hard, knotty, swollen, painful varicose veins of the leg, thigh and/or vulva that feel like they are stinging, bruised and sensitive to touch.

Lycopodium 12x Painful veins of the leg, thigh and vulva. Often the right side is affected, and then it might move to the left. Better for fresh air or warmth of bed. Worse between 4pm and 8pm. Worse for pressure and wearing tight clothes.

Pulsatilla 12x For painful, stinging conditions of the leg, thigh and/or foot. Poor circulation - limbs lain on become numb and cold. Worse for warmth. Better for fresh air.

support & resources

Dr Gowri Motha and her team of associates work at two venues in London.

Viveka
27a Queen's Terrace
St John's Wood
London, NW8 6EA
Tel: 020 8483 3788

The Jeyarani Centre
South Woodford
London, E18 2AL
Tel: 020 8530 1146

E-mail: gowrimotha@gentlebirthmethod.com
Website: www.gentlebirthmethod.com

'the jeyarani way' practitioner list

Dr Gowri Motha: Medical director and founder of the Jeyarani Way programmes.

Debbie Linger: Reflexologist, creative healer, Theta healer, Reiki healer, Bowen practitioner, hypnotherapist and PICT trained psychotherapist – teaches the Jeyarani Way Gentle Birth Method classes.

Kasia Ayub: Reflexologist, creative healer, Reiki healer and Bowen practitioner.

Marion Mckay: Reflexologist, creative healer, Theta healer, Reiki healer and Bowen practitioner.

Sherine Lovegrove: Reflexologist, creative healer, Theta healer, hypnotherapist and psychotherapist.

Carol Murray: Hypnotherapist, Theta healer and creative healer – teaches the Jeyarani Way Gentle Birth Method classes for couples and runs the self-hypnosis and Theta-healing classes for fertility enhancement.

Ali Cuthbert: Reflexologist, creative healer and Ayurvedic massage practitioner.

Dr Joya Das: Medical doctor in general practice and Theta healer.

Candida Hillman: Creative healer, colour light practitioner and massage practitioner – teaches the Jeyarani Way Gentle Birth Method self-hypnosis and visualization classes.

Vanessa Emery: Reflexologist, creative healer, massage therapist and Reiki healer.

Yvette Goh: Colour light practitioner and Reiki healer.

Lynne Howard: Clinical Homeopath – works with mothers and babies and advises on immunizations.

Sandra Bickmore: Pilates teacher, Bowen practitioner and personal trainer.

Practitioners at Viveka are dedicated to working with mothers and babies. Appointments can be made with consultant obstetricians, gynaecologists, paediatricians, clinical diagnostic services, cranial osteopaths, homeopaths, acupuncturists and healers. Please refer to the website (www.viveka.co.uk) for details.

useful contact details

Dr Palitha Serasinghe: Assistant Director and Principal Lecturer at
The College of Ayurveda (UK), 20 Annes Grove, Great Linford, Milton
Keynes, MK14 5DR.
Dr Serasinghe also consults and treats at the Jeyarani Centre, focussing
on pregnancy massage for birth preparation and post-natal recovery and
advising on fertility for couples.

HOMEOPATHIC PRACTITIONERS

Lynn Howard MCH RSHom: Tel: 020 7254 7821.
Felicity Fine MCH RSHom: Tel (at Viveka): 020 7483 3788.

NUTRITIONISTS

Marilyn Glenville and her team of experts consult at Viveka. For
appointments, call 020 7483 3788.

COLOUR LIGHT PRACTITIONERS

Pre- and post-natal colour light treatments for non-verbal trauma
resolution for mothers and babies.

Demari Armehlle Italiano: 32 Rogers House, Page Street, Pimlico,
London, SW1 4EX. Tel: 020 7821 1143, mobile: 07973 315950.

Kamla Deva: 14 Peter Street, Taunton, Somerset, TA2 7BZ. Tel: 01823
288 082, mobile: 07980 372776.

Yvette Goh: 32 Cleveland Road, London, E18 2AL. Mobile: 07944 250195.

Charaka Satyam: Troed-Y-Bryn, Alltwallis Road, Carmarthen, SA32 7DY. Tel: 01267 253213.

Elaine Swords: 275B Barlowmoor Road, Manchester, M21 7GH. Tel: 0161 881 2644.

CRANIO-SACRAL ASSOCIATES

For pre- and post-natal treatments for mothers and babies.

Thomas Attlee: Principal of the College of Cranio-sacral Therapy, 9 St George's Mews, Primrose Hill, London, NW1 8XE. Tel: 020 7586 0120.

Lynn Haller: Consults at Viveka. Tel: 020 7483 0099 (appointments).

Carla Lamkin: Consults at Viveka. Tel: 020 7483 0099 (appointments).

PILATES ASSOCIATES

Sandra Bickmore: Based in Essex, Sandra offers one-to-one training in her studio as well as group classes for pre- and post-natal recovery. Tel: 020 8501 4179, e-mail: corefit@btconnect.com

James de Silva: Based in St John's Wood, James offers personal one-to-one studio training. Tel: 07966 144442.

YOGA ASSOCIATES

Françoise Freedman: Founder of Birthlight pre- and post-natal yoga, and teacher of the Aquanatal programme for mothers and baby-swim programmes at Swiss Cottage, London. Website: www.birthlight.com.

Katy Appleton: Pre- and post-natal yoga. Website: www.appleyoga.com.

These are some useful websites to find out about classes in your area:

www.waterbabies.co.uk
www.aquatots.com
www.littledippers.co.uk
www.waternippers.com

For baby neoprene wetsuits and other useful baby swim products:
www.babyswimshop.co.uk
www.jojomamanbebe.co.uk

WATERBIRTH

Splashdown Water Birth Services: Offer seminars for midwives and doctors and for mothers and fathers on freedom in choice for birthing and parenting. Website: www.waterbirth.co.uk.

STRESS AND TRAUMA RESOLUTION IN INFANTS, CHILDREN AND ADULTS

Deirdre Youngs: Practitioner and teacher of Polarity Therapy and pre-natal and birth therapy, focusing on pregnancy/babies/children/families. Based in Norfolk, Deirdre offers Birth Process Workshops to assist adults in transforming birth trauma in the UK and abroad. Tel: 01263 761125, website: www.innercentre.org.

Chantek McNeilage: Cranio-sacral therapist, pre-natal and birth therapist and massage/bodywork (including infant massage). Based in Cambridge, Chantek supports babies, children and families, and facilitates Birth Process Workshops in the UK and Europe for adults wishing to resolve early life trauma. Tel: 01799 522516, e-mail: chantek@ntlworld.com.

Graham Kennedy: Based in Reading, Graham is a Cranio-sacral therapist and senior tutor at the Institute of Cranio-sacral Studies (tel: 0118 9863986, e-mail: admin@craniosacralstudies.co.uk) and a pre-natal and birth therapist specializing in helping babies, children and adults resolve early life stress and trauma. Website: www.internal-awareness.co.uk.

suppliers

In general, health food shops stock aromatherapy essential oils, Bach flower remedies, popular homeopathic remedies and nutritional supplements, including essential fats for mother and baby.

The Nutri Centre: Tel: 020 7436 5122, website: www.nutricentre.co.uk.
Planet Organic: Tel: 020 7221 7171, website: www.planetorganic.com.
G. Baldwin and Co. Herbalists: Tel: 020 7703 5550, website: www.baldwins.co.uk.
Ainsworth Homeopathic Pharmacy: Website: www.ainsworth.com.

The Jeyarani Centre provides teaching material for self help at home with products such as the Creative Healing postnatal toning home massage treatments:
The Baby Massage DVD
The Postnatal Pilates DVD
The Creative Healing for Fertility Enhacement Workshop DVD
Website: www.gentlebirthmethod.com.

TAPES AND CDS

Toning up after Birth 'The Jeyarani Way', Dr Gowri Motha. Postnatal visualization and deep relaxation to help you regain your pre-pregnant shape and tone and be more beautiful that ever before! Available on CD and tape.

Sleep Tape, Dr Gowri Motha. A general relaxation tape with specific mind–body conditioning suggestions to induce deep restful sleep. Can help you to go back to sleep quickly if awakened. Available on CD.

COT MOBILES

I particularly recommend the Symphony in Motion series which is battery-operated (rather than wind-up) and plays for 15-minute intervals. It is available from Mothercare, John Lewis, larger Boots stores, all major department stores and specialist baby shops and catalogues.

further reading

Gentle Birth Method, Dr Gowri Motha and Karen Swan MacLeod, Thorsons, London, 2004, ISBN 0-00-717684-8

Birth and Beyond, Dr Yehudi Gordon, Vermilion, London, 2002, ISBN 0-09-185694-9

Birth Without Violence, Frederick Leboyer, Mandarin, 1991, ISBN 0-7493-0642-4

Blooming Birth, Lucy Atkins and Julia Guderian, Collins, London, 2005, ISBN 0-00-718401-8

Bright Start, Dr Richard C. Woolfson, Hamlyn, London, 2003, ISBN 060060537X

Primal Health: Understanding the Critical Period between Conception and the First Birthday, Michel Odent, Clairview Books, 2002, ISBN 1902636333

Homeopathy for Pregnancy, Birth and Your Baby's First Year, Miranda Castro, St Martin's Griffin, 1993, ISBN 0-312-08809-4

Baby Minds: Brain-Building Games Your Baby Will Love, Linda Acredolo and Susan Goodwyn. Published by Bantam Books, 2000, ISBN 0-553-38030-3

Being with Babies: What Babies Are Teaching Us (booklets in 2 volumes),Wendy Anne McCarty, self-published, 2000 (available from www.wondrousbeginnings.com)

Bonding: Building the Foundation of Secure Attachment and Independence, Marshall Klaus, John Kennell and Phyllis Klaus, Addison-Wesley Publishing Company, 1995, ISBN 0-201-44198-5

From Conception to Crawling: Foundations for Developmental Movement, Annie Brook, self-published by author, 2001, ISBN 0-976-04491-9 (available from www.anniebrook.com)

Parenting from the Inside Out, Daniel Siegel and Mary Hartzell, Tarcher Putnam, New York, 2003, ISBN 1-58542-209-6

Reflexes, Learning and Behaviour, Sally Goddard, Fern Ridge Press, USA, 2002, ISBN 0-9615332-8-5 (available from www.inpp.org.uk)

The Aware Baby, Aletha Solter, Shining Star Press, California, Revised Edition 2001, ISBN 0-9613073-7-4

The Mind of Your Newborn Baby, David Chamberlain, North Atlantic Books, 1998, ISBN 1-55643-264-X

QUOTATIONS

The Red Tent, Anita Diamant, Pan, London, 2002

Perfume, Patrick Suskind, Penguin, London, 1987

index